KEEP IT SIMPLE

101 BEST
YOGA ASANAS
FOR HEALTH AND RELAXATION

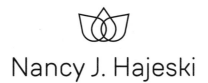

Nancy J. Hajeski

GENERAL DISCLAIMER

The contents of this book are intended to provide useful information to the general public. All materials, including text and images are for informational purposes only and are not a suitable substitute for medical diagnosis, advice, or treatment for specific medical conditions. All readers should seek expert medical care and consult their own physicians before commencing any regimen for any general or specific health issue. The author and publishers do not recommend or endorse specific treatments, procedures, advice, or other information found in this book and specifically disclaim all responsibility for any and all liability, loss, or risk, personal or otherwise, which is incurred as a consequence, directly or indirectly, of the use or application of any of the material in this publication.

President: Sean Moore
Production Director: Adam Moore
Editorial Director: Lisa Purcell
Author: Nancy J. Hajeski
Art Direction: Philippa Baile at OilOften Graphic Design, London. www.oiloften.co.uk
Design: Kate Williams at KatieLoveDesign Ltd.

Editor: Karen Lawrence

ISBN: 978-1-62669-148-3

Printed and bound in China

10 9 8 7 6 5 4 3 2 1

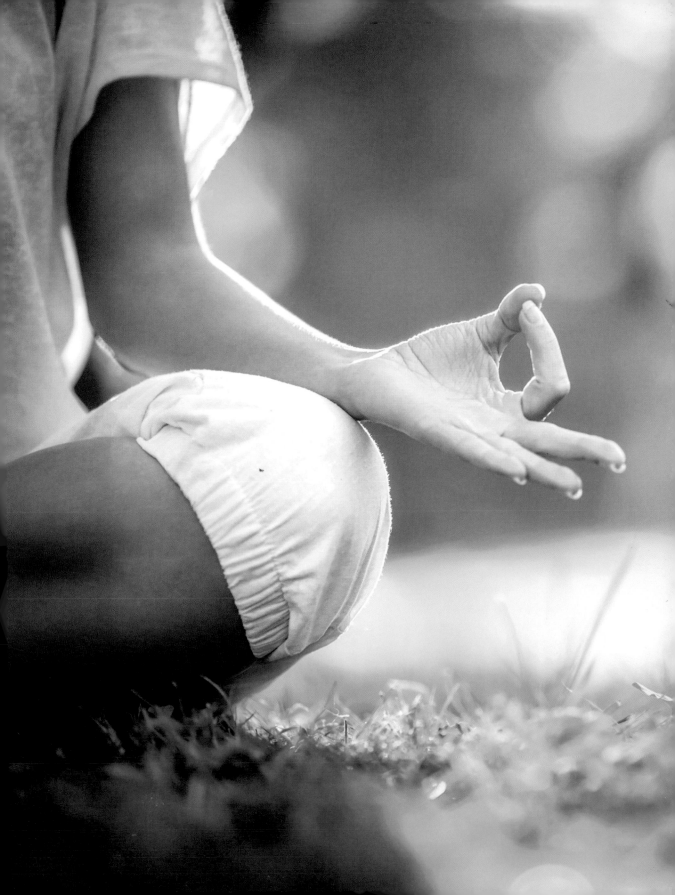

Contents

CHAPTER FIVE
Arm Supports

CHAPTER SIX
Backbends

CHAPTER SEVEN
Seated Forward Bends

CHAPTER EIGHT
Reclining Poses

GLOSSARY

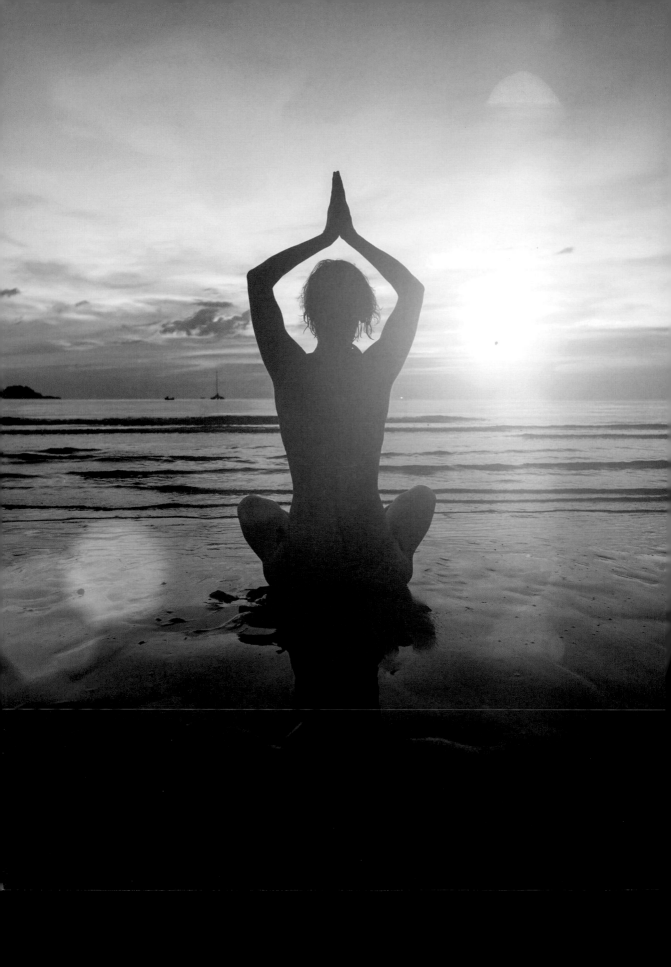

INTRODUCTION

Transform Your Life

In simple terms, yoga is a spiritual and ascetic discipline which incorporates the use of specific body postures to promote health and calmness. In America, nearly 20 million people practice it annually...and more than that number report an interest in pursuing it.

Although it is usually taught in a class, yoga is not about competition. Every student competes with only one person: themselves. Each pose is performed according to that individual's level of proficiency, with little pressure from without to work harder, go deeper, or "feel the burn." If an asana proves too taxing, the student can sink down into Child's Pose to rest and recuperate... without recrimination. The study of yoga is a very personal pursuit, which is one of its many charms.

Yoga is also the secret weapon of body builders who want to stay flexible; athletes who need to stretch deeply; and dancers, who require a way to unwind after the mental rigors of a performance.

BODY, MIND, SPIRIT

Some practitioners dismiss claims that yoga can also calm the mind, energize the thoughts, balance the psyche, and refresh the spirit. Conversely, many of those who study yoga, even novices, soon understand the truth of these claims. There is a reason that people who mediate often assume yoga poses to facilitate the body-mind connection. There is something about stretching the body and holding still as you breathe in measured beats that creates a powerful release of stressors, one that can be felt physically, mentally, and spiritually.

Be aware, however, that yoga done well, done properly, requires discipline. Even some beginner poses need to be worked up to gradually. Yet consider how therapeutic yoga can be for the office worker who slouches in a chair all day...or the computer tech who hunches over a keyboard...or the harried at-home parent whose stress levels are through the roof. Just take that first step, complete your first asana, and the benefits will quickly become clear. You will soon be taking classes to improve your technique and attempting sequences at home.

This book offers a primer covering 101 of the most popular foundation poses and the most versatile wellness-building asanas, which can be performed by novice and advanced student alike. Whether you are just starting out or are coming back to yoga and using the book like a refresher course, you will find a wealth of information here. Each entry includes step-by-step instructions, detailed photos, tips on finessing a pose, pitfalls to watch out for, and a variation or modification for each pose. Everything you need to begin a healthful, restorative journey.

STAY LIMBER, STAY BALANCED, STAY SERENE.

A Venerable History

Yoga has been practiced for millennia. At different times is has been valued as either a physical discipline or a path to mental and spiritual growth, and sometimes, as is true today, as both. Technically, yoga is considered a psychosomatic practice, where the physical benefits cannot be separated from the psychological. (So even if you don't exactly believe in the mental or spiritual aspects of yoga, you will still experience them.)

The timeline of yoga's evolution is classified into four categories— Vedic, Preclassical, Classical, and Postclassical—each era making its own contributions to the genesis of yoga as we encounter it in the present.

VEDIC YOGA

Yoga is believed to have originated in the Indus Valley within the Indus-Sarasvati civilization of India starting around 3,000 B.C. The yogis, or seers, of that time encouraged the union of the finite transitory self, or jiva, with the infinite eternal self, or Brahman— the Hindu term for god.

This early period takes it name from the Vedas, especially the Rig-Veda,

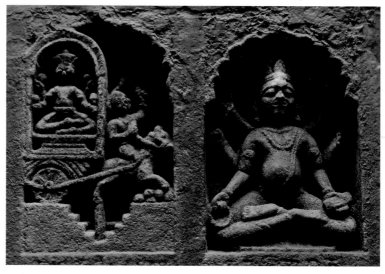

books of collected hymns that established many tenets of the Hindu religion. Vedic yoga focused on the broadening of the mind and extolled a quiet life spent close to nature.

PRE-CLASSICAL YOGA

This period lasted for approximately 2,000 years, up until around 200 AD. It coincided with the advent of the Upanishads, Hindu scriptures written in the Vedic tradition. This era produced many schools of thought, which offered numerous techniques for achieving the deep meditation needed to transcend the body and mind. Around 600 B.C., the Bhagavad Gita, a work that summarized many aspects of yoga, outlined three key paths: Karma, the path of generous action; Bhakti, the path of devotion; and Jnana, the path of knowledge.

CLASSICAL YOGA

From 200 B.C. to 400 A.D., a more systematic presentation of yoga developed. Called Sutras, these were brief statements, easily committed to memory, that were used to express complex ideas. In his second-century book, Yoga Sutras, sage Patanjali composed some of the most important ones, which are still studied

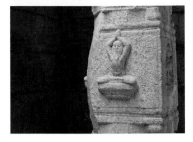

Yogi symbol on the column in the temple of India Hampi.

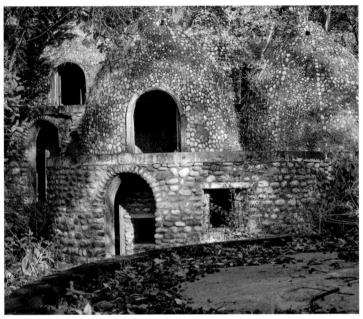

Meditation cells at the abandoned Maharishi Mahesh Yogi Ashram (Beatles Ashram).

and interpreted today. This book was the most translated Indian text during the medieval period, translated into 40 Indian languages. It disappeared for 700 years, and was then rediscovered late in the 19th century and again in the 20th century. It is considered one of the foundations of classical yoga philosophy.

POST-CLASSICAL YOGA

Yoga of this period differs from its predecessors—it teaches students to welcome reality rather than shun it, and to live in the moment. After centuries of study behind the "silk curtain," the practice of yoga finally found its way into the Western world in the early 1800s. Later in that century, a number of yogis toured Europe and America and became celebrities. Yet it was not until the 1930s that the practice of yoga was accepted as a form of exercise. By the middle of the 20th century, celebrated yogis like Maharishi Mahesh—who promoted Transcendental Meditation—and Swami Sivananda—who opened schools in Europe and America— were teaching and explaining the foundational beliefs of yoga. It was

Sivananda who formulated the Five Principles of Yoga: Savasana (relaxation), Asanas (exercise), Pranayama (breathing exercises), Diet, and Dhyana (positive thoughts) along with Meditation.

Currently, the study of yoga has become a global phenomenon— it is practiced by people from around the world, in all walks of life, and at all economic levels. (One of yoga's compelling features is that it requires no other equipment than a cushioned area on which to stand or sit.) Men, women, teens, children, even seniors, have fallen under its spell—and have seen their health, and mental outlooks, improve as a result.

Although yoga has evolved over the eons, many of its original concepts, ideals, customs, and positions have endured. And because yoga fosters a non-judgmental attitude, a wide variety of people feel welcomed within its culture.

Yoga Varieties

Numerous styles or variations of yoga have evolved over the passing centuries, and many of them are taught in modern yoga studios. Before committing yourself to classes in a particular discipline, it helps to have an overview of what each type of yoga involves. Try attending several different classes in order to discover which variations best suit your needs or taste. And keep an open mind...some aspect of a session you were hesitant about may actually end up appealing to you.

THE HATHA TRADITION

Hatha is a branch of yoga that dates back to the 11th century or possibly quite a bit earlier. Hatha translates from Sanskrit as "force," and it is known as the yoga of activity, incorporating as it does a system of physical techniques or postures, called asanas. During the early 20th century, the poses that comprised I latha yoga—some of them combined with gymnastic exercises—became very popular with fitness advocates. Hatha yoga was soon simply referred to as yoga.

VINYASA

This version of yoga is quite popular and is taught at most large studios and gyms. The term "vinyasa" refers to linking breathing with movement, The poses are frequently performed in sequences—the "vinyasa flow"—that can appear almost like a choreographed dance. Sessions may be accompanied by traditional music and soft lighting.

ASHTANGA

The name refers to the "eight limbs" mentioned in Patanjali's Yoga Sutras, and the discipline is often identified as traditional Indian yoga. Ashtanga synchronizes breath with movement as the student proceeds through a series of positions, or asanas. These postures are always performed in the same sequence: Sun Salutation A, Sun Salutation B, a standing sequence, and a closing sequence. The session is conducted without music, sometimes without any verbal input.

IYENGAR

Popularized in the West by Indian yogi B.K.S. Iyengar, this discipline emphasizes using breath control and props such as blankets, bolsters, blocks, and straps. It is taught without music

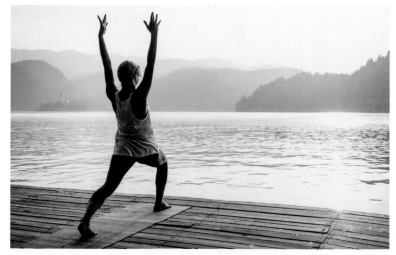

and occurs at a relatively slow pace meant to help students attain deeper postures.

BIKRIM
Introduced to California in the 1970s by Bikrim Choudhury, this form of yoga is comprised of 26 postures and two breathing exercises. Sometimes known as "hot yoga," Bikrim is practiced in a studio with the temperature set to 105 degrees Fahrenheit and with 40 percent humidity...and with a wall of mirrors so that students can frequently check the alignment of their asanas.

JIVAMUKTI
The name of this yoga variation translates to "liberated being." Not surprisingly, these classes appeal to students who seek a blend of the physical and spiritual—sessions may include chanting in Sanskrit, breath control, and asanas, along with a lesson or theme.

POWER YOGA
Although it is based on the traditional Hatha yoga poses, this discipline takes a more active approach. Asanas are performed more quickly, and with the addition of core exercises and upper body work. Sequences vary and there

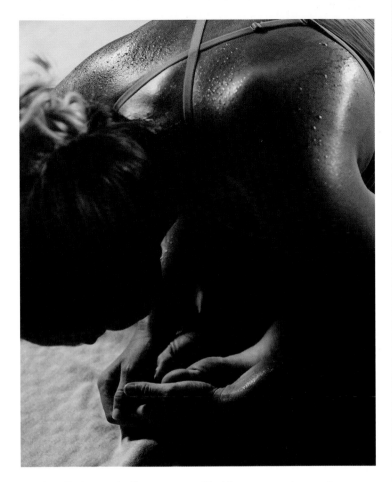

is often lively music. Some gyms offer Vinyasa as a type of Power yoga.

SIVANANDA
Brought to America by celebrated yogi Swami Vishnudevananda in the 1950s, this discipline is based on his five yogic principles: proper breathing, relaxation, diet, exercise, and positive thinking. The asanas used feature 12 basic postures along with Sun Salutations and Savasana, or Corpse Pose.

YIN AND YANG
Yin yoga is a passive variation that focuses on meditative poses that allow the body to remain comfortable without doing any strength work. Also called Taoist yoga, the asanas concentrate on elongating the connective tissues of the body. Yin is meant to compliment Yang yoga, which is an active, muscle-building form of yoga.

Clothing & Equipment

Yoga can be performed almost anywhere—in the office, in a hotel room, outdoors in a park, even while stopped in traffic. The two most likely places, however, are in a studio/gym setting or in your own home. Most beginners start out taking classes and then practice their poses at home. And, as with any new pursuit or pastime, some basic equipment is required.

WHAT TO WEAR

The study of yoga does not require an expensive wardrobe revamp. Loose, comfortable clothing—a pair of stretchy leggings and a cotton T-shirt for women or gym shorts and a tank top for men—should work fine. Once you commit to the practice, you may consider purchasing yoga pants, as well as moisture-wicking tops and shorts.

The one thing you will not need is expensive footgear. Yoga is typically performed barefoot. This is because your feet need to be in contact with the mat to form a stable foundation for poses (nerve endings in your soles signal your brain, allowing the body to determine proper balance and joint positions). Practicing barefoot also engages the smallest muscles in your feet, making them stronger and healthier.

TOOLS AND PROPS

First and foremost, you will need a yoga mat that meets several criteria. It should be light enough to carry to class, but sturdy enough to offer firm support. It should feel slightly sticky to provide some traction; look for one with a non-skid, gripping surface. The average-size mat (around 5.5'x 2') is fine for most people, but extra longs and extra wides are also available. Mats are typically 1/4" thick, but you can find thinner mats for travel or thicker mats to ease achy joint. If you prefer eco-friendly products, there are mats made of recycled materials and sustainable cork.

All you need for most classes is a mat, towel, and water bottle, but it's a good idea to own a few props...do you really want your head resting on the studio's yoga blocks? Props include yoga blocks, straps, and wedges, all helpful for attaining poses. (Towels can be used in place of straps and, when folded, in place of blocks.) Other aids include yoga balls, foam rollers, yoga wheels, bolsters, meditation pillows, yoga gloves, knee pads, and hand weights.

A SERENE HOME SPACE

You might enjoy setting up a small yoga studio at home. (Consider that with a dedicated area, you are more likely to practice.) All you need is a relatively quiet space away from the bustle of family life. Equip your sanctuary with a wall mirror, a yoga mat, a basket for props, and a side table for your towel and water. You can increase the ambiance with a fan, wind chimes, plants, Asian wall hangings and artwork, incense, and music.

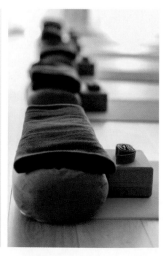

Breath Control & Hand Positions

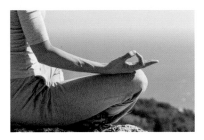

BEATHING FOR RELEASE

Pranayama is the Hatha practice of yogic breath control. The term translates as "suspension of breath," and, indeed, in early yoga culture it was intended to make "the mind swoon." Modern pranayama focuses on synchronizing the breath with one's movement during and between asanas. Research indicates that the techniques employed during pranayama can be beneficial to several stress-related disorders, including anxiety and mild depression.

Pranayama is practiced using a number of rejuvenating and calming exercises that oxygenate your lungs and help link your body and mind. They are best performed in sets of five to 10 repetitions while in a seated position.

Samavrtti ("same action") calms the mind and fosters a sense of balance. In this exercise you will observe any breathing irregularities, then transition into a slower and more even breath. To achieve the same, or equal, action in your breathing, inhale for four counts, and then exhale for four counts.

Ujjayi ("victorious breath") increases internal heat, tones the organs, improves mental focus, and eases stress. It has been called "ocean breath" due to the sound it makes passing through the narrowed throat passage. Breathing evenly, constrict your epiglottis at the rear of your throat, close your mouth as you breath through your nose, and listen for the hiss.

Sithali ("cooling breath") comforts and cools the body Unlike most other pranayama exercises, inhalation occurs through the mouth. Curl the sides of your tongue up, and stick it slightly out of your mouth. Inhale through the hollow of your tongue. Hold your breath briefly, close your mouth, and exhale through your nose.

Anuloma Viloma ("alternate nostril breathing") can lower the heart rate and ease tension. Begin with the Vishnu Mudra, with your index and middle fingers of your right hand curled down. Place your thumb on the outside of your right nostril, and inhale through your left nostril, keeping your mouth closed. Then close your left nostril with your ring finger, and hold momentarily. Lift your thumb, and exhale out of your right nostril. Then repeat with your right nostril.

MUDRAS

Mudras are the traditional yogic hand positions that often accompany asanas. They are said to cause a reflex reaction in a certain part of the brain; replicating the position directs a flow of energy to that spot.

Vishnu Mudra: Curl your index and middle fingers downward, while keeping your ring finger and pinky together and pointed outward. Use this mudra during Anuloma Viloma.

Gyan Mudra: Press the tips of the index finger and thumb together. This position represents knowledge and expansion.

Shuni Mudra: Press the tips of the middle finger and thumb together. This mudra represents patience and discernment.

Surya Ravi Mudra: Press the tips of your ring finger and thumb together. This position represents courage and responsibility.

Prayer Mudra: Press the palms of both hands together. This mudra is believed to balance the positive (male) and negative (female) sides of the body.

Venus Lock: Interlace the fingers of both hands, with the right pinky down for women,and the left pinky down for men. This mudra represents sexuality.

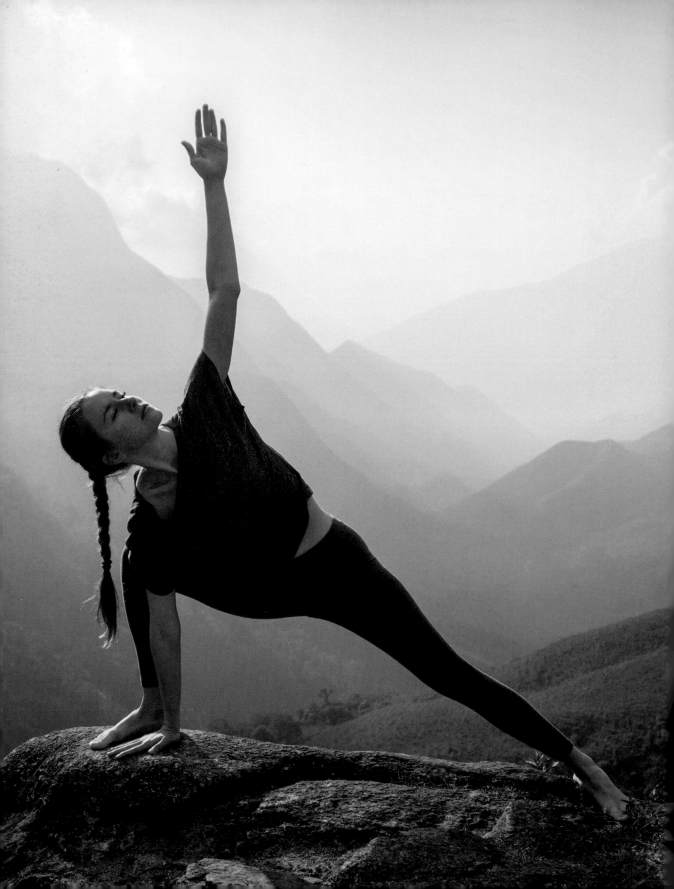

CHAPTER ONE
Standing Poses

Standing poses form the foundation of modern yoga and are typically performed at the beginning of a yoga session. They work to energize the body, build stamina, and strengthen your arms, shoulders, torso, hips, legs, and feet. They also improve your body's stability, balance, and posture...and can furthermore give indications of where weakness or instability lies. Once you have mastered the standing poses, you will find that your body falls naturally into graceful alignment.

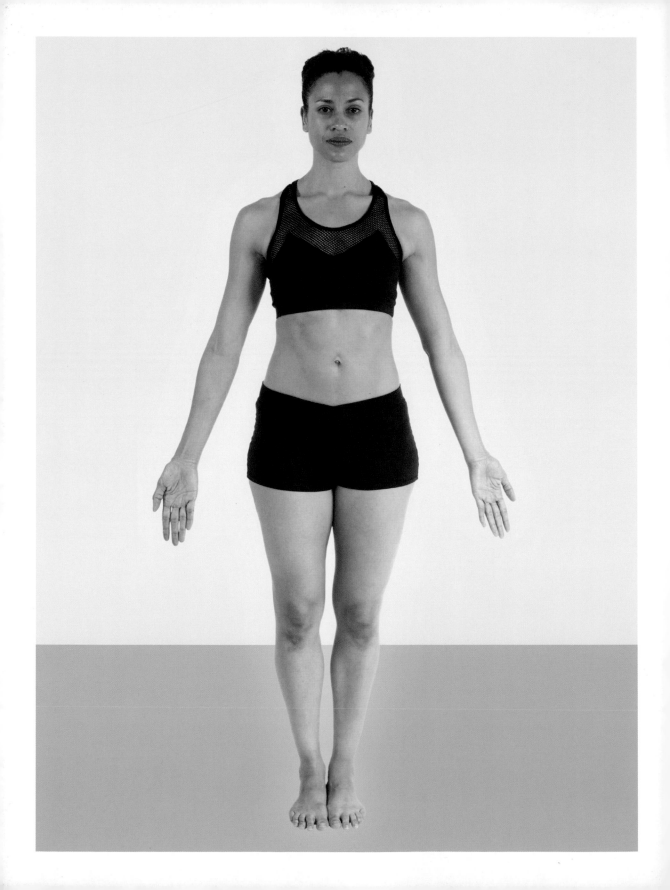

BEGINNER
INTERMEDIATE
ADVANCED

Mountain Pose

This beginner pose, also known by its Sanskrit name, TADASANA, is the starting position for many other standing poses. It is not described in the medieval hatha yoga texts, making it a relatively recent asana. It works to strengthen the thighs, knees, and ankles and to improve posture, groundedness, stability, and confidence.

FIND YOUR FORM

To make sure that you feel grounded during this pose press all four corners of each foot into the floor. For the most effective results, also remember to keep your arm, leg, and torso muscles engaged.

BE CAREFUL OF...

Avoid this pose if you suffer from headaches, insomnia, or low blood pressure.

STEPS

1. Stand tall with your back straight and feet together or slightly apart. Raise your toes up and separate them before returning them to the mat.
2. Active your legs by drawing your thigh muscles up and in toward your midline.
3. Raise your ribs and lengthen your spine, but don't sway your back. Tuck in your tailbone—think of your pelvis as a bowl holding water.
4. Activate your arms by stretching down through your fingertips, palms facing out. Draw your upper arms back and down, with your chest open and your palms now facing inward. Hold for four to six breaths.

VARIATION

Prop Aid Touch: If you feel wobbly, place a yoga block between your thighs to bring your feet to hip-width apart.

BEGINNER

INTERMEDIATE

ADVANCED

Upward Salute Pose

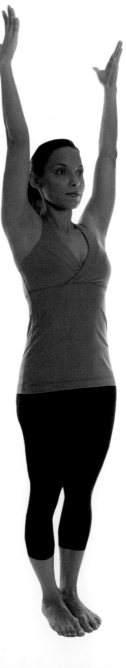

FIND YOUR FORM

Make sure your arms are straight overhead and parallel to each other. Soften any tension that remains in your shoulders.

BE CAREFUL OF...

If your shoulders feel tight, you can position your overhead arms into a wider "Y" formation. Don't hunch your shoulders up near your ears.

STEPS

1. While standing in Mountain Pose (p.16), stretch down through your fingertips.
2. Externally rotate your arms and raise them overhead, shoulder-width apart, palm facing palm.
3. Stretch up into your fingertips as you press your feet into the mat.
4. Gaze forward, and hold for three to five breaths.

Like Mountain Pose, Upward Salute appears deceptively simple, but it can be challenging to do correctly. Also known as URDHVA HASTASANA in Sanskrit, this pose is part of the venerable Sun Salutation sequences. It stretches the whole body, targeting the torso—the biceps, the obliques, and the abdominals—as it improves balance.

VARIATIONS

Arms Extended Pose: From Upward Salute, bring your arms down until they are level with your shoulders, palms facing up.
Backward Bend: From Upward Salute, carefully sway your arms back beyond the line of your shoulders.

INTERMEDIATE

ADVANCED

Tree Pose

FIND YOUR FORM

When first attempting this pose, you might want to use a wall as a brace for your back.

BE CAREFUL OF...

Avoid letting your hips jut out; keep them both squared forward.

STEPS

1. Begin in Mountain Pose (p.16) with your arms at your sides.
2. Shift your weight onto the left side of your body, keeping the inner left foot firmly on the floor.
3. Bend your right knee and place the sole of your right foot against the inside of your left thigh. The position of your legs should resemble the number 4.
4. Keep your hips facing forward and centered in a neutral position.
5. Once you feel balanced, bring your palms together in front of your heart, as if in prayer. Hold for five to eight breaths and then repeat with the opposite leg.

VARIATION

Extended Tree Pose: For an increased challenge, while in Tree Pose raise both arms over your head, keeping your elbows straight, and press your palms together. Hold for four to seven breaths.

Also known as VRIKASANA, this pose is one of the simplest externally rotated balancing poses. It strengthens the vertebral column, thighs, and calves, as well as stretching the thorax, groin, and inner thighs. Tree Pose has long been a part of the yoga tradition, dating back to medieval hatha yoga.

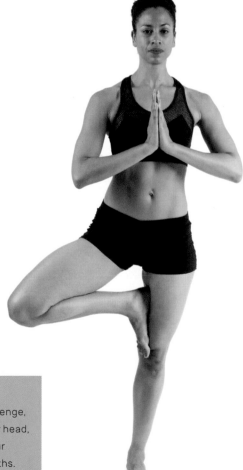

INTERMEDIATE

ADVANCED

Palm Tree Pose

FIND YOUR FORM

During the entire pose make sure your eyes remain slightly above horizon level.

BE CAREFUL OF...

Women in the early stages of pregnancy may benefit from the gentle stretching of the abdomen, but they should avoid the pose after the first trimester.

Also known as TADASANA, this pose stretches the entire body, including the arms, chest, abdomen, spine, and legs. It is useful as a warm-up or after performing inverted poses as the means for redistributing blood throughout the body. You may experience a sense of mental and physical balance during this pose, especially if you close your eyes.

STEPS

1. Stand upright with hands relaxed and legs slightly apart
2. Raise your hands straight over your head and interlock your fingers with the palms facing up. Adjust your gaze to just above the horizon.
3. On a deep inhale, stretch your arms, shoulders, and chest upwards while keeping your elbows bent to create a gentle curve. Avoid arching your back.
4. Stretch the entire body from toes to head to hands.
5. Hold for three to six breaths.

VARIATION

Palm Tree Side Bend: While your hands are extended overhead with fingers interlaced, lean your torso to the left from your hips, hold for several breaths, come upright, and then lean to the right.

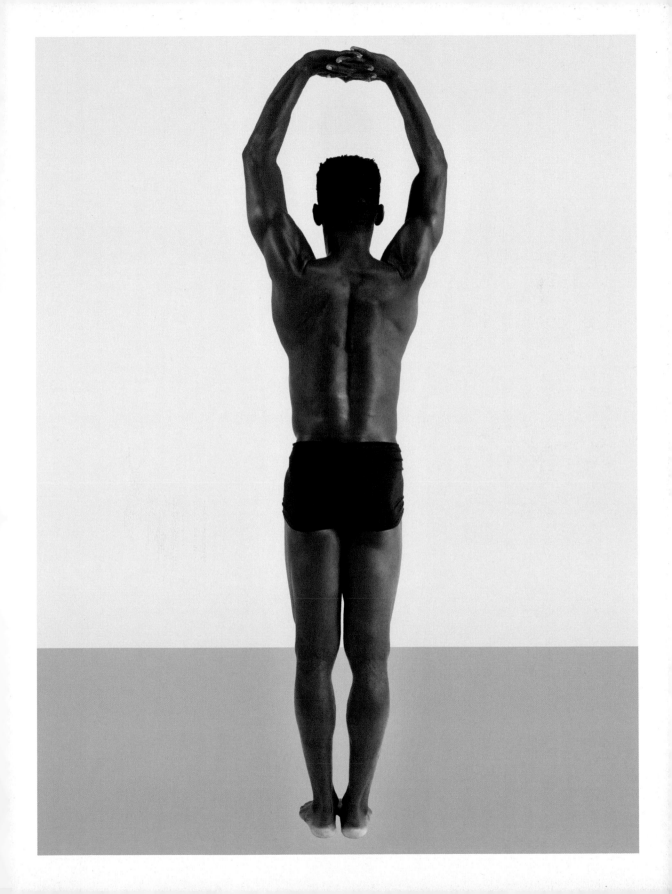

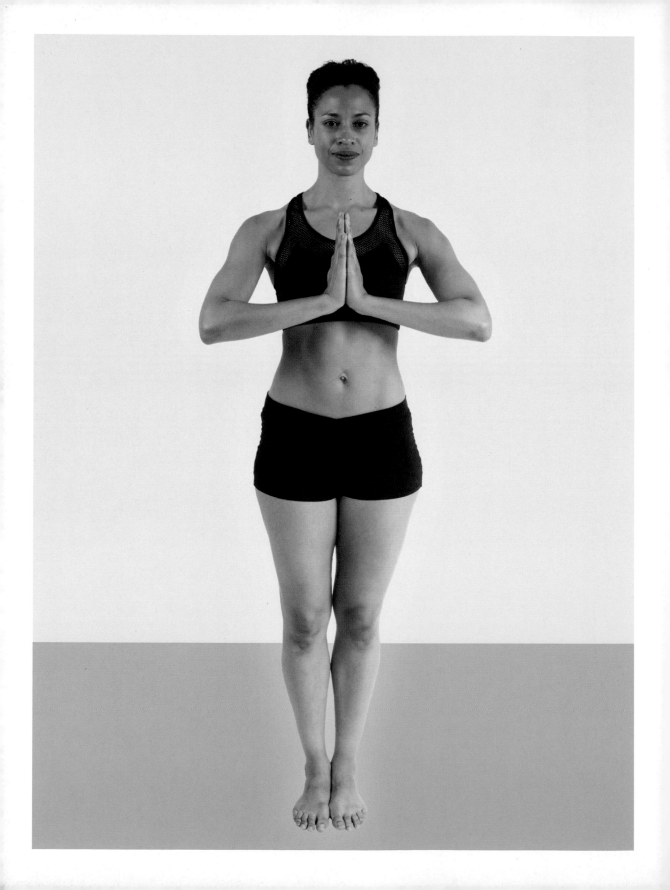

BEGINNER

INTERMEDIATE

ADVANCED

Prayer Pose

FIND YOUR FORM

Stand up straight, with your shoulders stacked over your hips, hips stacked over knees, and knees in line with your feet.

BE CAREFUL OF...

Try not to overtuck your pelvis or push your ribs forward.

Also known as PRANAMASANA, this restorative centering pose is often used as part of the Sun Salutation sequence or as a transition between other poses. The palms-together prayer position, called Anjali Mudra, completes an energy circuit between the hands and the heart, harmonizing the two. It is often used to accompany the greeting "Namaste."

STEPS

1. Begin by standing in Mountain Pose (p.16).
2. Press your palms together, moving your hands into prayer position and lowering them to your heart. Keep your neck relaxed, your chin parallel to the floor, and your gaze forward. Avoid arching your back.
3. Hold for five to eight breaths.

VARIATION

Reverse Prayer: Bring your arms behind your back, fingers pointing down. Press your palms together and rotate your hands inward so that your fingers point up.

BEGINNER
INTERMEDIATE
ADVANCED

Standing Side Bend

FIND YOUR FORM

Soften any tightness in your shoulders, and keep them from hunching up near your ears.

BE CAREFUL OF...

Do not let your torso bend forward or backward as you lean to the right. Avoid this pose if you have neck, shoulder, or lower back issues.

This pose may not look challenging, but it requires concentration and flexibility. It can be used as a warm-up before a stretching routine or performing any asanas that require flexibility. It stretches the upper and middle back as well as the abdominals and obliques.

STEPS

1. Start out in Mountain Pose (p.16) with your hands at your sides, palms turned inward against your thighs.
2. On an inhale, raise your left arm out to the side and then lift it straight above your head, fingers outstretched.
3. Keeping your raised arm straight, lean your upper torso to the right, consciously extending the left side of your body.
4. Keep your hips and knees squared as you lean. Your head and neck should be in neutral position.
5. Hold for four to six breaths before repeating on the other side.

VARIATION

Prop Aids: For an easier version of this stretch, grasp a yoga strap or resistance band taut in your upraised hands and spread them wider than shoulder-width apart. Lean to the side until you feel a stretching sensation.

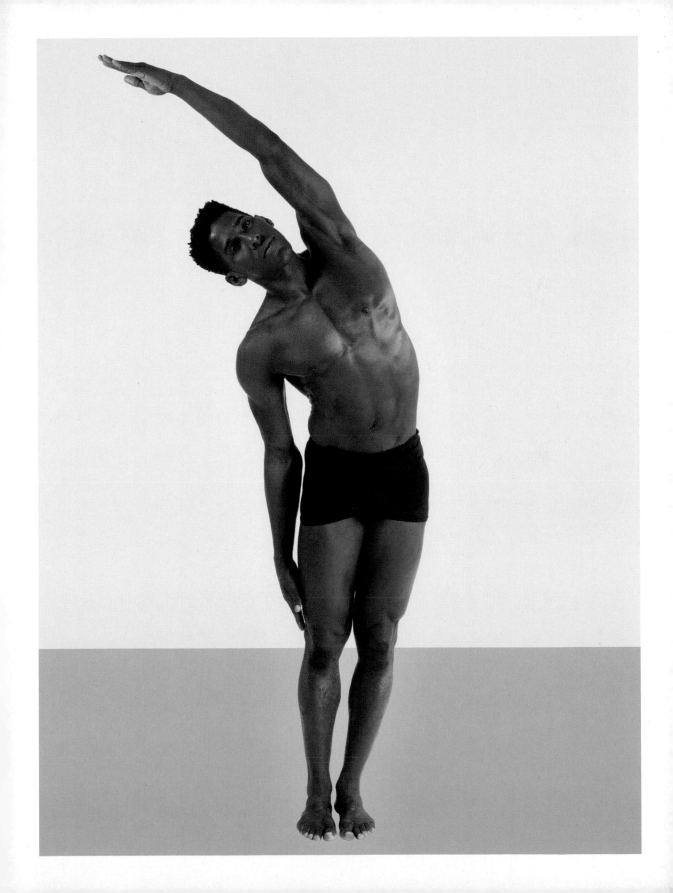

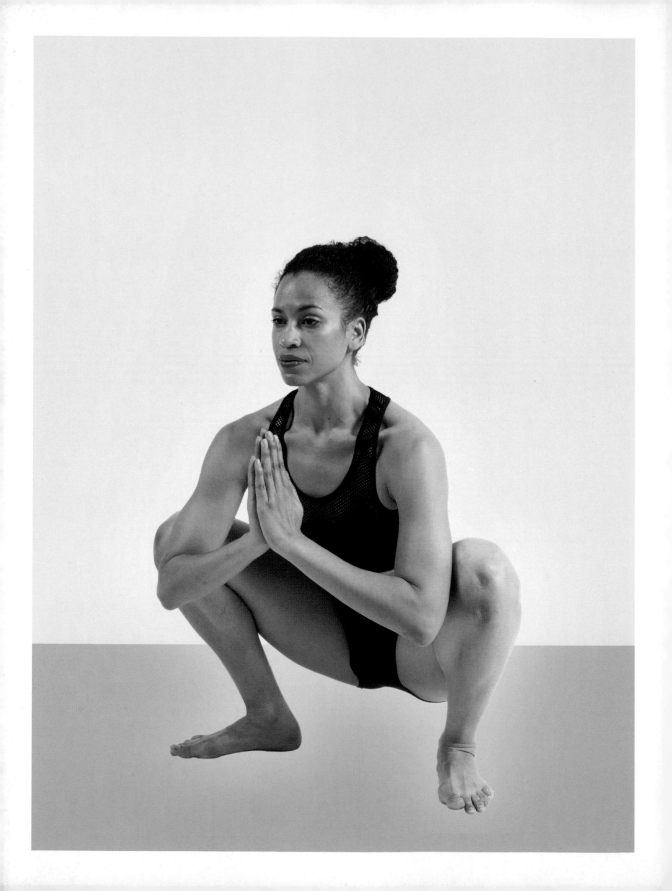

BEGINNER

INTERMEDIATE

ADVANCED

Garland Pose

FIND YOUR FORM

As you squat, use your elbows to create gentle pressure on your knees, spreading them even wider and increasing the inner thigh stretch.

BE CAREFUL OF...

Watch out that you don't round your shoulders forward. Avoid this pose if you have lower-back or knee issues.

MALASANA is a beginner pose that targets the inner thighs, opening up the hips and thigh joints. It also stretches the back, hips, groin, and ankles. This squatting pose is particularly beneficial to pregnant woman and is safe to be performed by them throughout all three trimesters.

STEPS

1. Begin in Mountain Pose (p.16) facing the front short edge of your mat.
2. Place your feet farther than shoulder-width apart.
3. Bend your knees deeply, lowering yourself into a squatting position until your hips are lower than your knees.
4. Press your palms together in front of your heart in prayer position as you broaden across your collarbones. Hold for three to six breaths.

VARIATION

Prop Support: If you find it difficult to keep your heels on the ground, place a folded blanket or towel under them.

BEGINNER

INTERMEDIATE

ADVANCED

Gate Pose

FIND YOUR FORM

As you reach down toward your toes, be sure to keep your arm straight. Keep your chin off your chest.

BE CAREFUL OF...

Avoid this pose if you have recent or chronic knee, hip, or shoulder issues.

Also called PARIGHASANA in Sanskrit, this beginner, kneeling side bend stretches the vertebral column, the hamstrings, and the intercostal muscles that connect the ribs, which improves the breathing process. Try this pose as a prep for Triangle Pose and Extended Side Angle Pose.

STEPS

1. Kneel facing the short side of the mat with the knees hip-width apart. Extend the left leg out straight to the side, with the toes flat on the mat; keep your right knee under your right hip.
2. Inhale and bring the right arm up to the ceiling and place the left hand, palm down, on the left shin.
3. Exhale as you bring the right arm beside the ear as you contract the left side of your torso and lean to the left. Slide your left arm along your shin, reaching toward your toes.
4. Press out with the right hip as you press down into your foot and knee.
5. Feel your chest open as you hold the pose for three to six breaths. Return to kneeling position and repeat with the other leg.

VARIATION

Prop Aid: To ease tight leg joints, place a folded blanket under the kneeling knee.

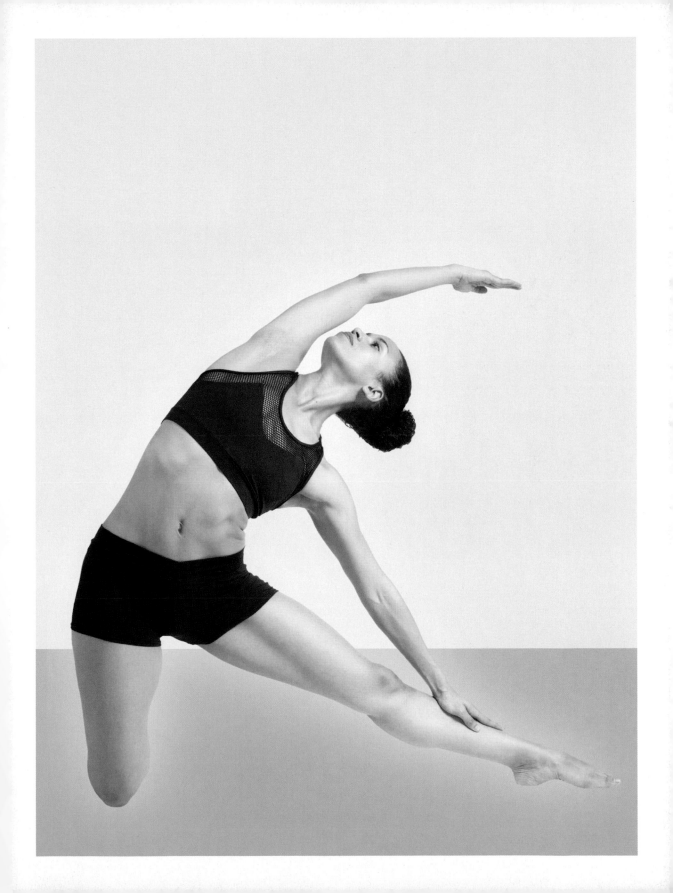

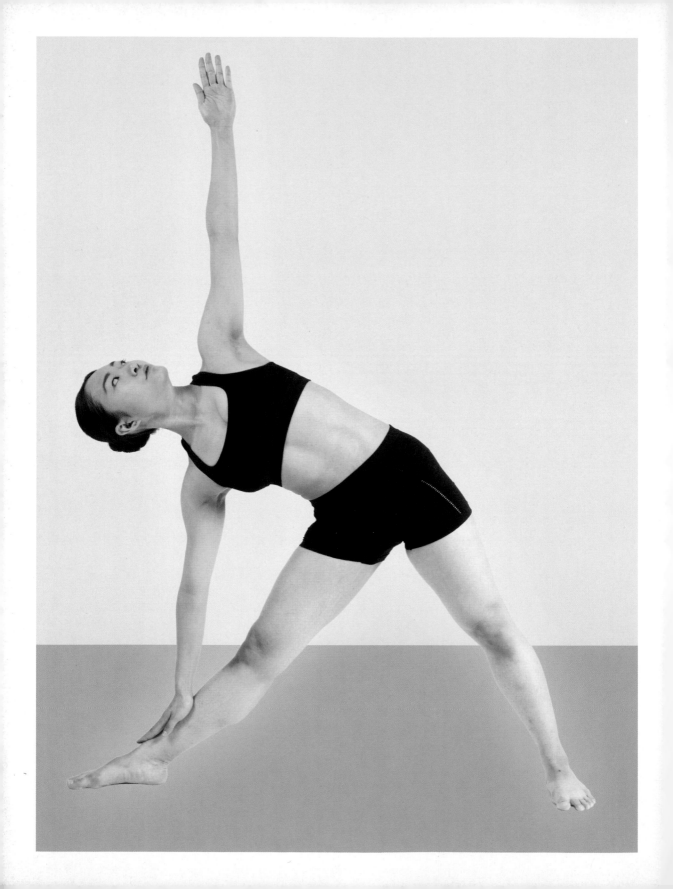

BEGINNER

BEGINNER

INTERMEDIATE

ADVANCED

Triangle Pose

FIND YOUR FORM

Keep your leading knee tight and aligned with the center of your foot, shin, and thigh; keep your back heel pressed to the floor during the bend.

BE CAREFUL OF...

Do not perform this pose if you have high or low blood pressure, a headache, or neck issues.

This pose, called TRIKONASANA in Sanskrit, is excellent for relieving neck and back tension and can also help to trim and tone your waist. It stretches the thighs, hips, knees, ankles, hamstrings, calves, shoulders, chest, and spine, and opens the groin. It is also beneficial for easing the symptoms of menopause and for stimulating digestion.

STEPS

1. Stand with your feet about three feet apart, with your right foot angled at 90 degrees and your left foot facing the front of the mat.
2. Raise both arms out to the side and parallel to the floor, palms down. Bend over to your right side and reach down so that your right hand is touching your lower shin or ankle and your left arm raised above you.
3. Gently twist your spine and torso to the back as your arms extend away from each other; your gaze should be fixed on your raised thumb.
4. Make sure you tuck your tailbone in as you try to get your whole body into one plane.
5. Hold this position for three to five breaths, and then inhale as you return to a standing position. Repeat on the other side.

VARIATION
Extended Triangle: To increase the effect of the stretch, widen your stance and reach past your lower shin and press your palm to the floor.

BEGINNER

INTERMEDIATE

ADVANCED

Horse Pose

FIND YOUR FORM

Keep your abdominals tucked in and your knees soft. Seek to move with graceful control.

BE CAREFUL OF...

Avoid twisting to the side, arching your back, or hunching forward. Do not perform this pose if you suffer from hip or knee issues.

This beginner pose, which targets the hamstrings, hips, knees, and quads, is also known as a Sumo Squat or Plié Squat—or VATAYANASANA in Sanskirt. Horse pose boosts energy while it strengthens hip adductors and improves sense of balance and lateral movement.

STEPS

1. Begin standing in Mountain Pose (p.16); step your legs out so that your heels are positioned beyond your hips.
2. Turn your heels in and toes out, but not to the point where you feel discomfort.
3. Inhale and raise your arms overhead, forming prayer hands.
4. Exhale and bend your knees until your thighs are as close to perpendicular with the floor as possible. At the same time bring your pressed palms down to your chest at heart level. Bring your shoulder blades down and hold for three to six breaths.

VARIATION

Horse Pose Palms Up: From Horse Pose raise your arm up to shoulder height with a slight curve in your elbows and palms facing up.

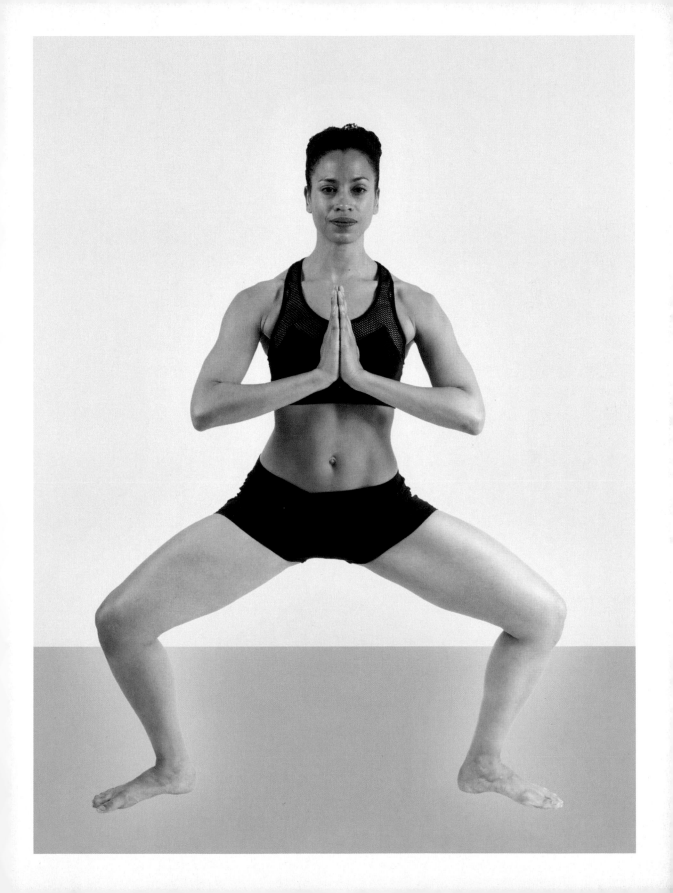

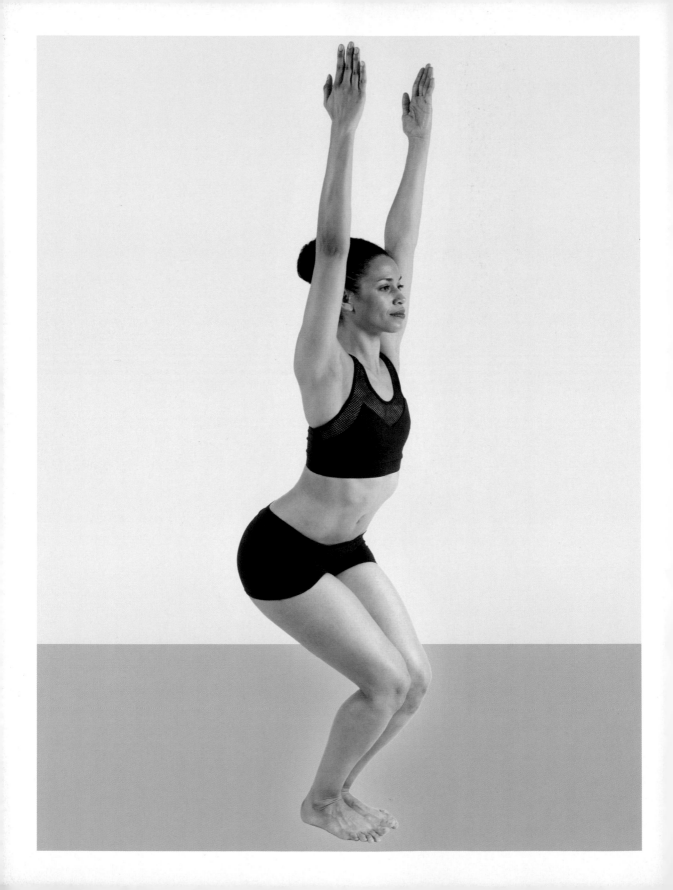

BEGINNER

INTERMEDIATE

ADVANCED

Chair Pose

FIND YOUR FORM

Draw your tailbone down as your roll your inner thighs toward the floor.

BE CAREFUL OF...

Avoid overarching your back or letting your knees knock.

This beginner pose, also called Awkward Pose and UTKATASANA in Sanskrit, asks the student to hinge at the ankles, hips, and knees and requires full body strength to maintain it. Eventually, once you are practicing longer holds, you will notice improvement in your leg and upper-body strength.

STEPS

1. Begin by standing in Mountain Pose (p,16). Inhale and bring your arms into Upward Salute (p.18), reaching above your head with your arms parallel.
2. As you reach upward, rotate your arms inward, so that your palms are facing each other.
3. Make sure your inner thighs, knees and ankles are touching as you exhale and bend your knees.
4. Shift your weight to your heels, draw your hips back, and position your knees slightly behind your toes. Hold for four to six breaths.

VARIATION

Calf on Knee Chair Pose: To add a balance challenge to the pose, rest the outer calf of either leg above the opposite knee as you maintain correct form with your body and arms.

Revolved Chair Pose

FIND YOUR FORM

Keep your pressed hands centered on your chest. Create a small hollow in your upper back as your broaden your collarbones.

BE CAREFUL OF...

Do not allow your shoulders to round as you twist. Avoid this pose if you have knee or back issues or are pregnant.

This side twist beginner pose, called PARIVRTTA UTKATASANA in Sanskrit, focuses on the back, lower body, and obliques. It helps to strengthen thighs, buttocks, ankles, and arms, while stretching the spine, the side muscles, and the abdomen. It is recommended for stimulating digestion and elimination.

STEPS

1. Start in Chair Pose (p.34) with your arms parallel over your head, palms facing, and your knees in a deep bend.
2. Inhale as you bring you hands to the front of your chest in prayer position, palms together.
3. Exhale and twist your upper torso so that it faces to the right, keeping your hips square.
4. Bring your left elbow down and hook it over your right knee. The right elbow should be pointed to the ceiling.
5. Inhale and lengthen your spine while drawing your navel in toward your spine. Swivel your head, and bring your gaze to the ceiling.
6. Hold for three to five breaths before switching sides and repeating.

VARIATION

Supported Revolved Chair Pose: To really open the chest, bring your lower arm down, and place your fingertips on the ground as you raise the upper arm above your shoulder, fingers extended.

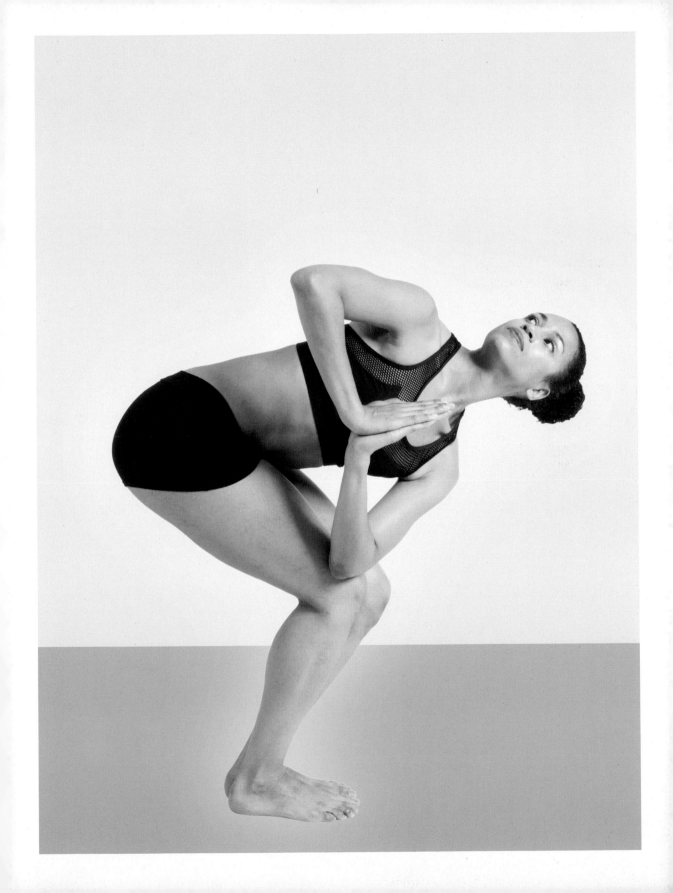

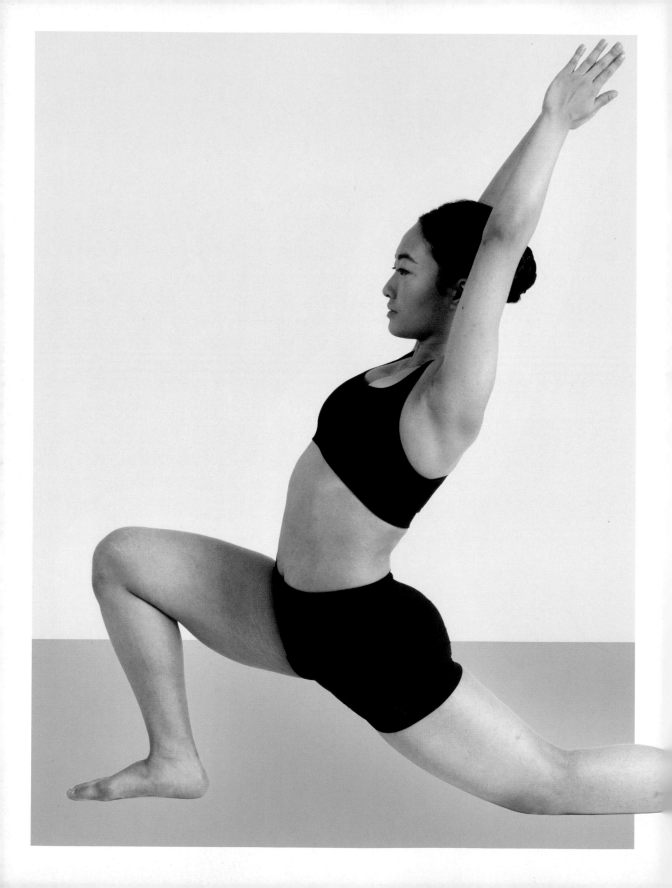

Low Lunge

FIND YOUR FORM

Be sure that your forward knee is positioned above your shin and ankle. You can deepen the stretch by shifting your pelvis forward.

BE CAREFUL OF...

Don't let your front ribs jut forward. Avoid this pose if you suffer from lower-back issues or have a knee injury.

The upright backbend known as ANJANEYASANA or Equestrian Pose can be found in many yoga sequences. It effectively stretches the shoulders, chest, arms, and lower body, strengthens thighs and hip abductors, and improves balance and stability.

STEPS

1. Begin in Downward Facing Dog (p. 192). On an exhale, step your right foot forward between your outstretched hands.
2. Lower your left knee onto the floor with the top of your foot on the mat, Slide your leg back until you feel the stretch in your upper thigh and groin.
3. Bring your torso upright with your hands relaxed at your sides; inhale and sweep your arms out to the sides and then overhead, fingers pointing to the ceiling.
4. Tuck your tailbone in as you raise your pubis toward your navel.
5. Hold for three to six breaths, then fold down into Downward Dog, and repeat with the other leg.

VARIATION

Prop Aid: If you feel pain in your kneeling knee, place a folded blanket under it.

BEGINNER

INTERMEDIATE

ADVANCED

High Lunge

FIND YOUR FORM

Keep the back of your neck long as you gaze forward. Internally roll the inner thigh of the straight leg toward the ceiling

BE CAREFUL OF...

Do not position your knee over your toes, or you may risk injuring the knee.

Avoid this pose if you suffer from knee pain or issues.

This beginner lunge, PRASARITA PADOTTANASANA, is often found in yoga sequences as a transition pose from forward bends or arm supports. It stretches the hip flexors, shoulders, and chest while it strengthens the thighs and increases your sense of balance.

STEPS

1. Begin in Downward Facing Dog (p.192) and step your left foot forward between your hands until your knee and shin are lined up with your ankle.
2. Balance on your fingertips as you press your left heel into the floor, and square your hips to the front of the mat.
3. Stretch your right leg behind you, with your weight on the ball of the foot, the toes curled forward.
4. Elongate your torso from your crown to your back knee.
5. Hold for three to six breaths before returning to Downward Dog and repeating with the other leg.

VARIATION

Prop Aid: If your back rounds as you reach for the floor, try placing your hands on yoga blocks.

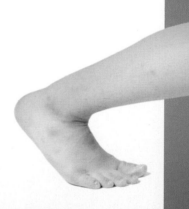

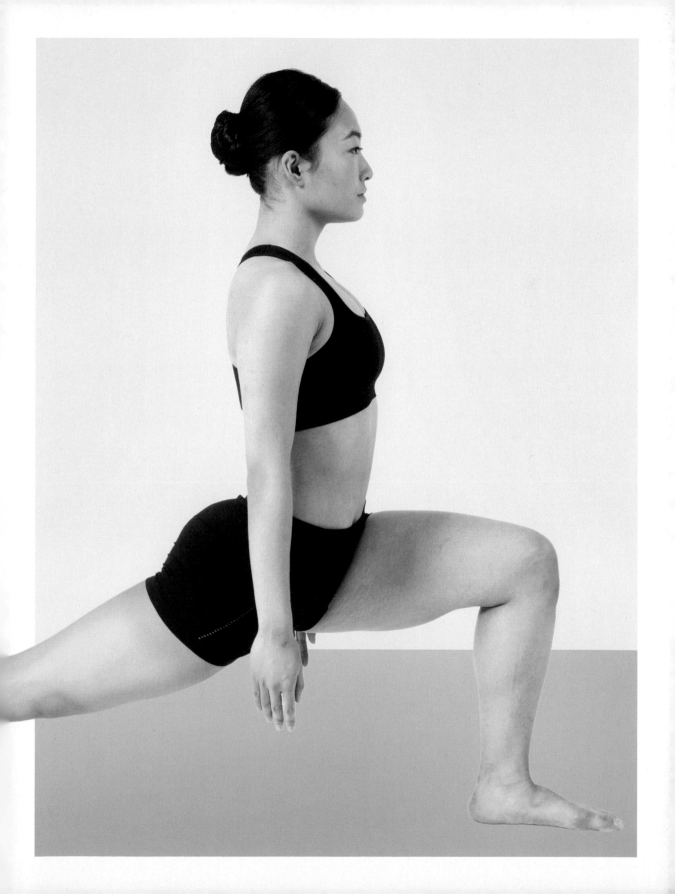

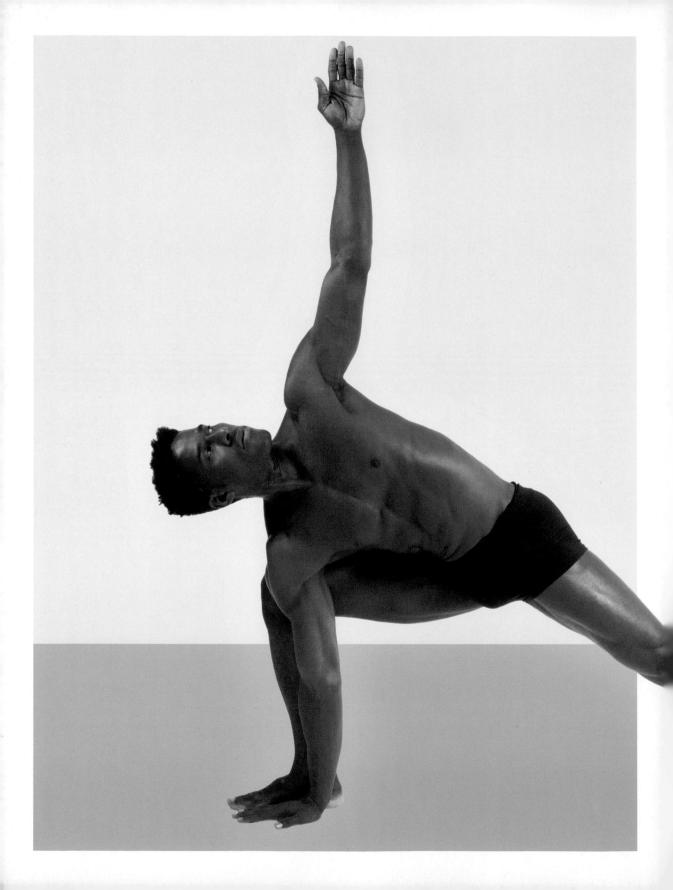

BEGINNER
INTERMEDIATE
ADVANCED

Side Angle Pose

FIND YOUR FORM

Make sure you bend from your hips not your waist. Keep your forward knee aligned with the center of your shin and foot.

BE CAREFUL OF...

If you feel wobbly, brace your back against a wall. Avoid this pose if you have high or low blood pressure or neck problems.

By building up your strength and felxibility, this useful beginner pose, called PARSVAKONASANA in Sanskrit, makes an excellent preparation for the more demanding standing poses. It also tones the core, opens the hips, and is useful for easing the symptoms of menopause.

STEPS

1. Stand in the middle of your mat in Mountain Pose (p.16) hands on hips.
2. Step your feet apart about three or four feet. Position your right toes to face the upper-right corner of the mat and make sure your right heel is aligned with your left arch.
3. Bend your right knee until it is directly over your ankle.
4. Press the outer edge of your left foot into the mat and allow energy to draw upward to your hip as you internally rotate the back leg to keep it neutral.
5. Extend both arms out to the side, palms down, until they are parallel to the floor.
6. Bend your torso toward your right knee, and reach down inside the right calf toward the floor. Stretch your left arm upward, fingers reaching for the ceiling.

VARIATION

Deep Stretch Side Angle: To raise the difficulty level, try reaching out to the side with your raised arm and bringing your torso down toward your thigh until you feel a deep-seated side stretch.

BEGINNER

INTERMEDIATE

ADVANCED

Eagle Pose

FIND YOUR FORM

Make sure your hips do not twist to either side but remain squared to the front.

BE CAREFUL OF...

Do not attempt this pose if you suffer from knee or groin injuries.

This demanding beginner pose, known as GARUDASANA, not only improves your balance, it also requires stamina and focus. Along with stretching the hips and buttocks and releasing stress in the back, it strengthens the thighs, knees, and ankles. The pose is also recommended for enhancing concentration.

STEPS

1. Begin in Chair Pose (p.34) and extend your arms out to the sides.
2. Shift your weight onto your right heel as you bend your left knee and bring your left thigh up over your right thigh. Attempt to wrap your left toes around the back of your right calf.
3. Bend your elbows and raise your arms in front of you. Hook your right elbow beneath your left elbow, entwine your forearms, and bring your palms together, fingers facing up.
4. Find a fixed object to gaze at as you hold the pose for three to five breaths; repeat with the opposite leg and arm.

VARIATIONS

Supported Eagle Pose: If you feel wobbly, place your raised foot on the ground outside the standing foot.

Bending Eagle Pose: To raise the ante, from Eagle Pose bend forward from your hips and place your elbows on your knees. Let your upper back round forward.

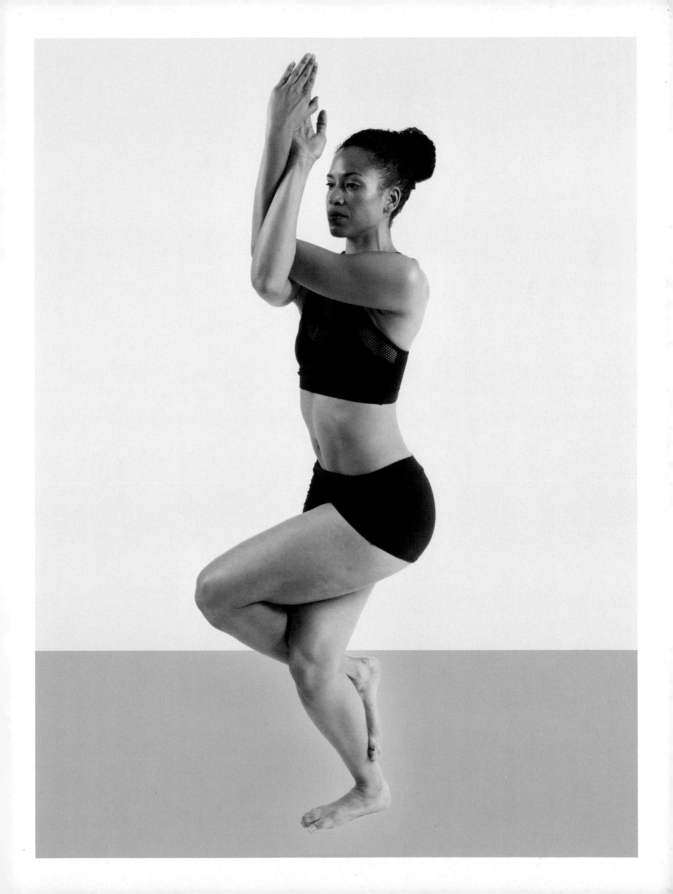

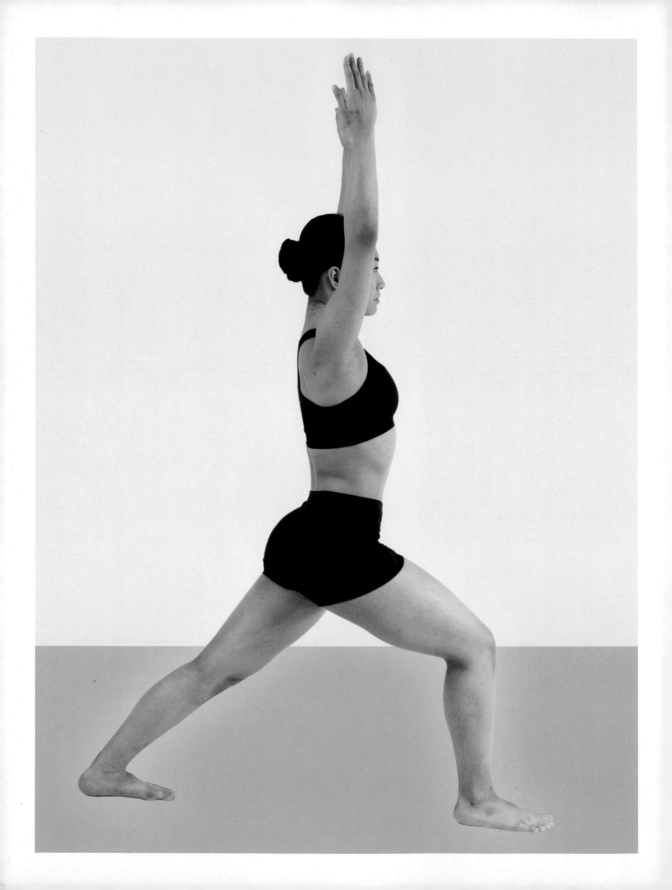

Warrior I Pose

FIND YOUR FORM

Remember to keep the bent knee directly above the ankle and the hips squared forward. Create healthy tension by stretching up with your arms as you ground down with your feet

BE CAREFUL OF...

Avoid twisting the knee of the straight leg. Do not perform this pose if you have knee, lower-back, or shoulder problems.

The Warrior Poses are a set of dynamic, challenging positions that require strength, stamina, and flexibility. Warrior Pose I, also called VIRABHADRASANA I, will help make you stronger in your shoulders, arms, thighs, calves, and ankles, and improve your confidence.

STEPS

1. Begin in Mountain Pose (p.16) in the center of the mat with your hands on your hips. Walk your legs apart about three feet, right foot to the front.
2. Turn your left foot out around 45 degrees until the toes are facing the left corner of the mat. Make sure both feet are in heel-to-heel alignment.
3. Bend your right leg as you inhale, and press all four corner of the foot into the mat. Press the outer edge of the left foot into the mat, and draw energy up through the leg to the hip.
4. Elongate your torso as you draw more upright, and bring your shoulder blades together. Reach your arms forward, and sweep them up over your head, palms facing each other.
5. Hold for two to five breaths or as long as is comfortable.

VARIATION

Deep Warrior: To deepen the pose, place your palms together overhead, gently arch your back, and gaze upward at the ceiling.

INTERMEDIATE
ADVANCED

Crescent Lunge

FIND YOUR FORM

Your upper body and raised arms should form a straight line, and your shoulders should be above your hips.

BE CAREFUL OF...

Try not to twist the knee of the back leg. Avoid this pose if you have knee, shoulder, or lower-back problems.

Although this pose is similar to Warrior I, and bears the same Sanskrit name, it creates a different dynamic in the rear leg because the heel is raised rather than flat on the floor. Like the Warrior Poses, this asana also increases your stamina.

STEPS

1. Begin standing in Mountain Pose (p.16) in the center of the mat with your hands on your hips.
2. Step your right foot three to four feet from your left foot so that it is facing the front of the mat. Raise your left foot onto the ball of the foot and press down into the mat.
3. Keep your left leg straight as you bend your right leg so that the knee is in line with your ankle.
4. Extend your upper torso and draw your navel toward your spine as you lift your arms straight above your head. Push energy up through your outstretched fingertips.
5. Externally rotate both arms with the palms facing each other. Hold the pose for three to six breaths before switching to the opposite leg.

VARIATION
Free Hands: While in Crescent Lunge, you can face your hands forward or curl them into claws.

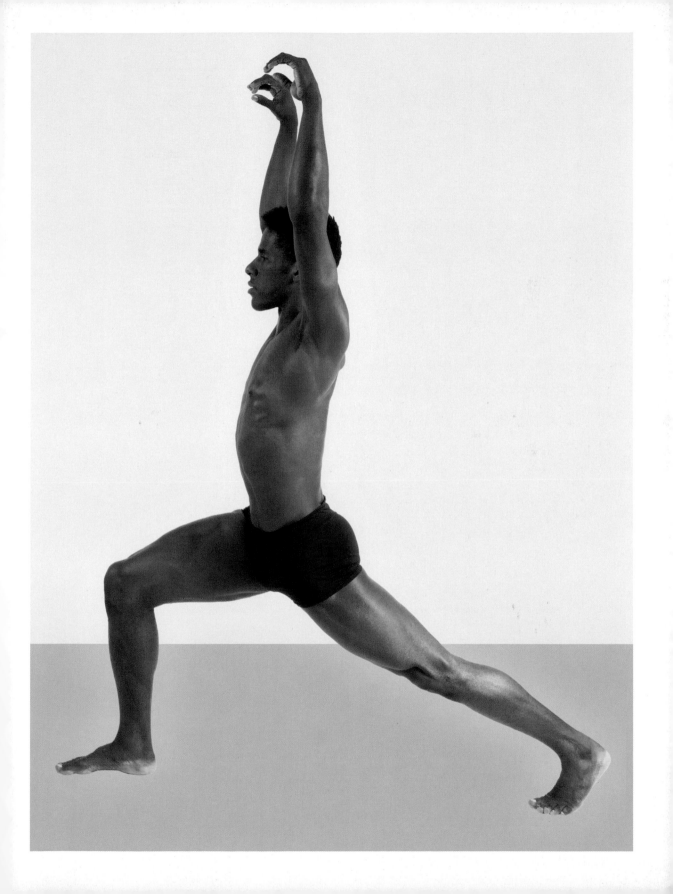

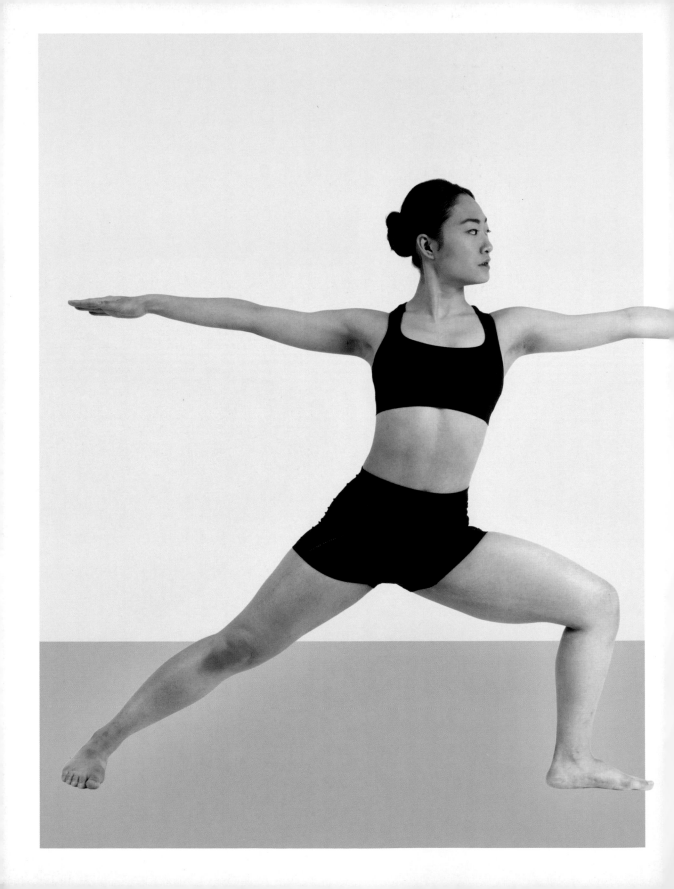

BEGINNER
INTERMEDIATE
ADVANCED

Warrior II Pose

In spite of its number, this pose is often approached before Warrior I. Also known as VIRABHADRASANA II, this asana serves to open the hips and stretches the shoulders, chest, and groin, as well as being a foundation position for a number of other poses.

FIND YOUR FORM

Be sure to keep your shoulders directly above your hips. Avoid this pose if you have shoulder, lower-back, or knee issues.

BE CAREFUL OF...

Do not arch your lower back or lean over your bent knee.

STEPS

1. Position yourself in the middle of your mat in Mountain Pose (p.16) hands on hips.
2. Step your feet apart about three or four feet. Position your left toes to face the upper-left corner of the mat and walk your foot until both feet are in heel-to-heel alignment.
3. Bend your left knee until it is directly over your ankle as you continue to press all four corners of your left foot into the mat.
4. Press the outer edge of your right foot into the mat and let energy draw upward to your hip as you internally rotate the back leg to keep it neutral.
5. Extend both arms out to the side, palms down, until they are parallel to the floor. Hold for three to five breaths; repeat with other side.

VARIATION

Arms Akimbo: For a less strenuous version, place your hands on your hips while maintaining torso and leg position.

BEGINNER
INTERMEDIATE
ADVANCED

Half Moon Pose

FIND YOUR FORM

You may gaze at your lowered hand, your raised hand, or to the side. It helps to immagine that your raised, flexed foot is pressing into a wall behind you.

BE CAREFUL OF...

Do not allow the knee of your supporting leg to twist out of alignment or your supporting foot to turn in. Avoid this pose if you have shoulder, neck, or knee problems or if you suffer from diarrhea, headaches, or high or low blood pressure.

This intermediate pose allows you to really open your hips and work on your balance and coordination. ARDHA CHANDRASANA stretches the torso, arms, and spine while strengthening the thighs and ankles. It can also been used to stimulate digestion and elimination.

STEPS

1. Begin in Extended Triangle Pose (p. 30 Variation) with your left hand or fingertips placed on the floor or on your shin. Gaze down at your left foot as you bring the other hand to your hip.
2. Shift more weight onto your left leg as you bring your right foot in about a foot.
3. Keeping your left hand down, slowly straighten your left leg, opening your thighs.
4. Raise your extended right leg to hip height, keeping it in neutral position, ankle flexed.
5. Find your center of balance, and raise your right arm straight up from the shoulder, opening your chest and collarbones. Hold for three to five breaths before repeating on the other side.

VARIATION

Block Aid: If you have trouble straightening your raised leg in this pose, try placing your lower hand on a yoga block. You can make the block taller by resting it on its side.

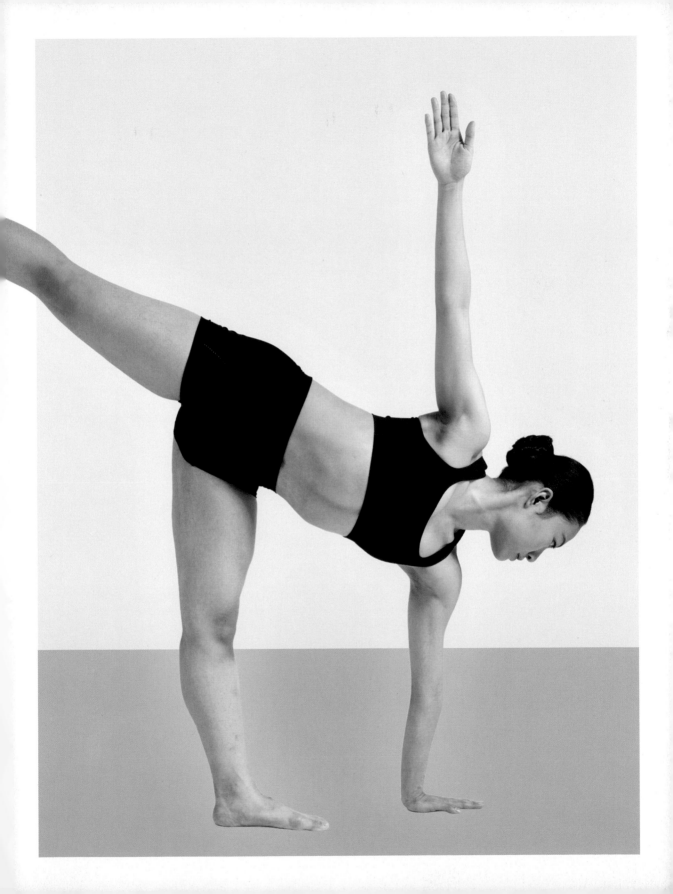

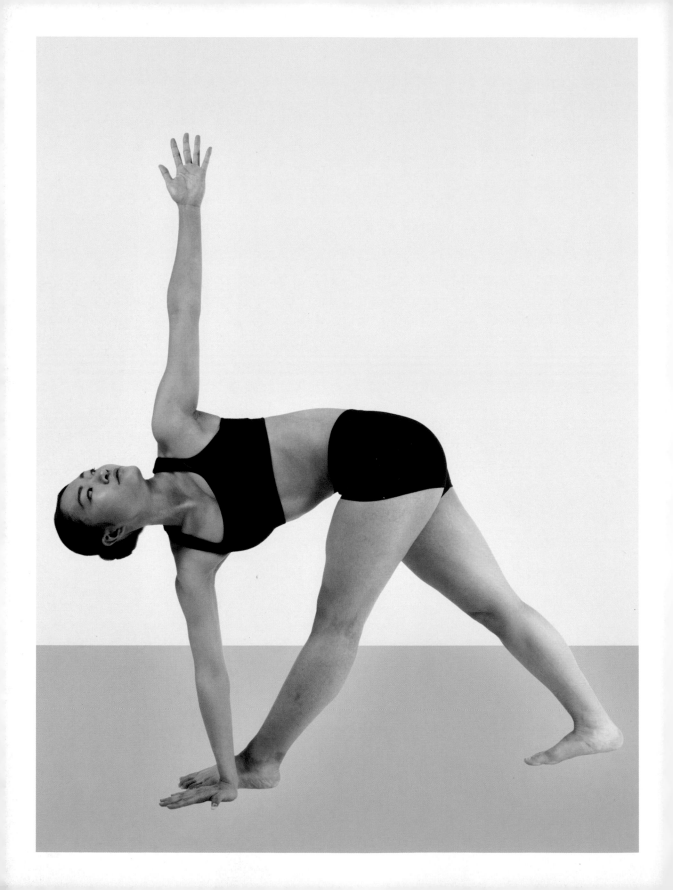

BEGINNER
INTERMEDIATE
ADVANCED

Revolved Triangle Pose

FIND YOUR FORM

Make sure to keep your arms and legs straight in this pose; if your hamstrings feel tight, slide your advanced foot even closer to the front of the mat.

BE CAREFUL OF...

Do not round your spine as you hold this pose. Avoid it if you have diarrhea, headache, high or low blood pressure, neck problems, or are pregnant.

This intermediate pose, called PARIVRTTA TRIKONASANA, draws on your hamstring and spine flexibility and also makes a good prep pose for forward bends and twists.. It is useful for strengthening your thighs and core and for improving your sense of balance. You may also want to try this pose as a digestion aid.

STEPS

1. Stand in the middle of the mat in Mountain Pose (p.16) with your hands on your hips and step your legs about three or four feet apart.
2. Turn your right foot 45 degrees so that the toes are facing the upper right corner of the mat. Bring your heels into alignment and then press down on the mat to ground your feet.
3. Inhale and extend your left arm above you, creating length along your left side; then hinge down as you twist your torso to the left, keeping your back flat.
4. Place your right hand on the mat on the outside of your left foot. Reach your left arm up toward the ceiling, opening your chest and collarbones. Hold for four to six breaths.
5. Exhale and twist the right side of your torso to the left as you gaze up at your raised thumb. Hold for three to five breaths before repeating on the opposite side.

VARIATION

Prop Aid: If you have difficult reaching your hand to the floor, place it on a yoga block positioned on the outside of your forward foot.

BEGINNER

INTERMEDIATE

ADVANCED

Extended Side Angle Pose

FIND YOUR FORM

Try to create a straight line from your rear leg to your upward-reaching arm. Open your hip by pressing the bent knee into the lowered arm.

BE CAREFUL OF...

Do not crunch your lower ribs or allow your shoulders to round forward as you bend. Avoid this pose if you have diarrhea or a headache, if you have high or low blood pressure, or suffer from shoulder or neck issues.

This intermediate pose, known as UTTHITA PARSVAKONASANA, is especially beneficial for stretching the muscles along the sides of the body—the quads, shoulders, obliques, chest, and hip adductors, as well as the hamstrings and buttocks. It also strengthens the core, hips, knees, and ankles.

STEPS

1. Begin in Mountain Pose (p.16) standing in the center of the mat. Step your legs three to four feet apart. Bend your left knee, and angle your left foot 90 degrees and shift your right foot in slightly. Your left heel should align with the arch of your right foot.
2. Internally rotate your right thigh while keeping the leg straight, and press your pinkie toe to the mat.
3. Raise your arms straight out from the shoulders parallel to the floor.
4. Exhale as you bend your torso to the left until your left hand touches the floor on the outside of your left foot. Inhale as you reach your right arm up toward the ceiling, fingers outstretched.
5. Rotate your arm as you bring it alongside your ear with the palm facing down. Fix your gaze on the underside of your extended arm. Hold for three to six breaths before repeating on the other side.

VARIATIONS

Block Aid: If you find it hard to touch your hand to the floor, place a yoga block on the outside of your forward foot.

Bound Version: For a real challenge, wrap your lower arm around your extended thigh, reaching back, and wrap your upper arm behind your back...and then join your hands together.

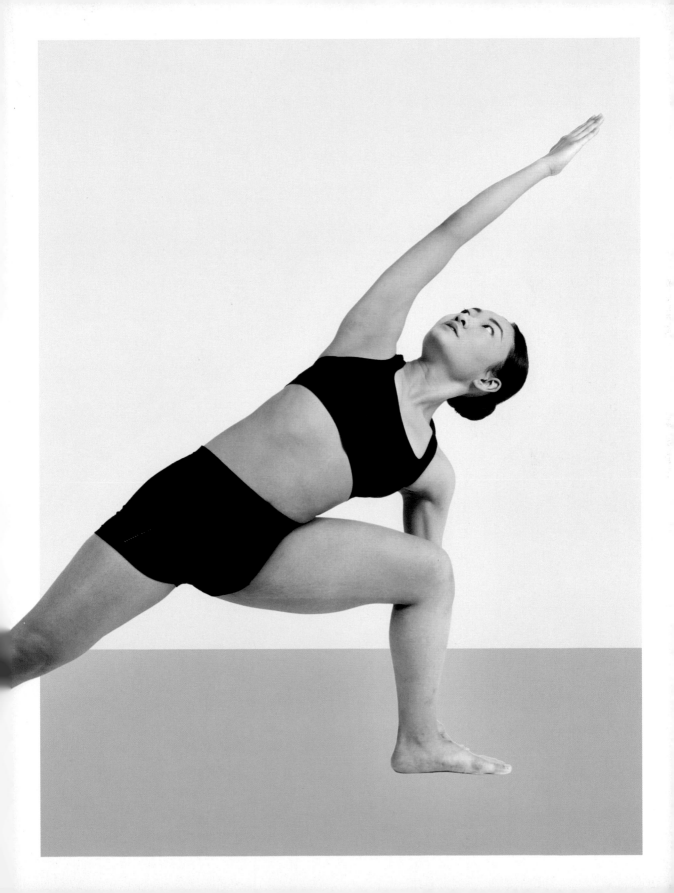

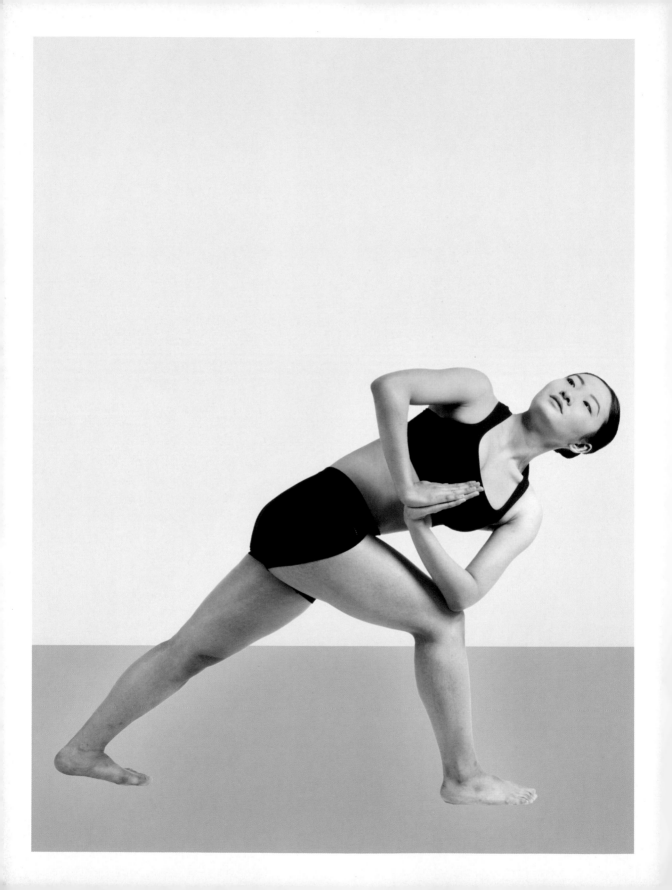

BEGINNER

INTERMEDIATE

ADVANCED

Revolved Extended Side Angle Pose

This intermediate deep-twisting pose, known as PARIVRTTA PARSVAKONASANA in Sanskrit, stretches the hips, arms, torso, groin, and spine. Use it to strengthen the thighs and ankles and to aid digestion and ease lower-back pain.

FIND YOUR FORM

Ground yourself by pressing the pinkie toe and edge of your rear foot to the mat. Your your front knee should be facing forward and aligned with your center toes.

BE CAREFUL OF...

Avoid this pose if you have diarrhea or a headache, if you suffer from high or low blood pressure, or have shoulder, knee, or neck issues.

STEPS

1. Begin in Mountain Pose (p.16) standing in the middle of the mat. Step your feet out three to four feet wide and turn your left toes inward at 45 degrees. Make sure your heels are aligned.
2. As you press your palms together in prayer position over your heart, bend your right knee so that your thigh is as close to parallel to the floor as possible. Keep your left leg straight out behind you with the thigh tight.
3. Twist your torso to face right and place your left elbow on the outer side of your right thigh near your knee; keep your hips squared. Press elbow to knee and knee to elbow for a deeper stretch.
4. Turn your gaze toward the right-hand back corner of the room. Hold for three to five breaths before repeating on the other side.

VARIATION

Arm Extension: For an equal challenge, raise your upper arm in line with your body and alongside your ear, and place the hand of your lower arm on the floor at the outer edge of your advanced foot.

BEGINNER

INTERMEDIATE

ADVANCED

Extended Hand to Big Toe Pose

This intermediate pose, UTTHITA HASTA PANDANGUSTHASANA, strengthens the legs and ankles, as well as stretching the back of the legs and opening the hips and groin. The pose requires you to stay focused on the supporting leg while you find your proper balance.

FIND YOUR FORM

Concentrate on elongating your torso, creating additional space between your breastbone and your pubic bone. It is also more important to elongate your spine than to straighten your extended leg.

BE CAREFUL OF...

Watch out that you don't elevate the hip on the side of the raised leg. Keep them level with the floor and facing forward. Avoid this pose if you have ankle, foot, or lower-back issues.

STEPS

1. Start in Mountain Pose (p. 16) and shift your weight onto your left foot, pressing all four corners into the ground to keep you steady.
2. Raise you left leg, grasp your left instep, bend your left knee up toward your torso.
3. Slide your fingers onto your toes and grasp your big toe with your thumb and forefinger curled around it. Rest your left hand on your left hip.
4. Exhale and slowly extend your right leg, gradually straightening it as you flex your extended foot. Keep your hips squared and your gaze ahead of you.
5. Hold for three to five breaths before repeating on the other side.

VARIATIONS

Side Swing: For a more effective stretch, at Step 4 swing your leg out to the side while keeping a two-finger hold on your toe.

Balance Test: Challenge your sense of balance by bringing your free hand out to the side and following that hand with your gaze.

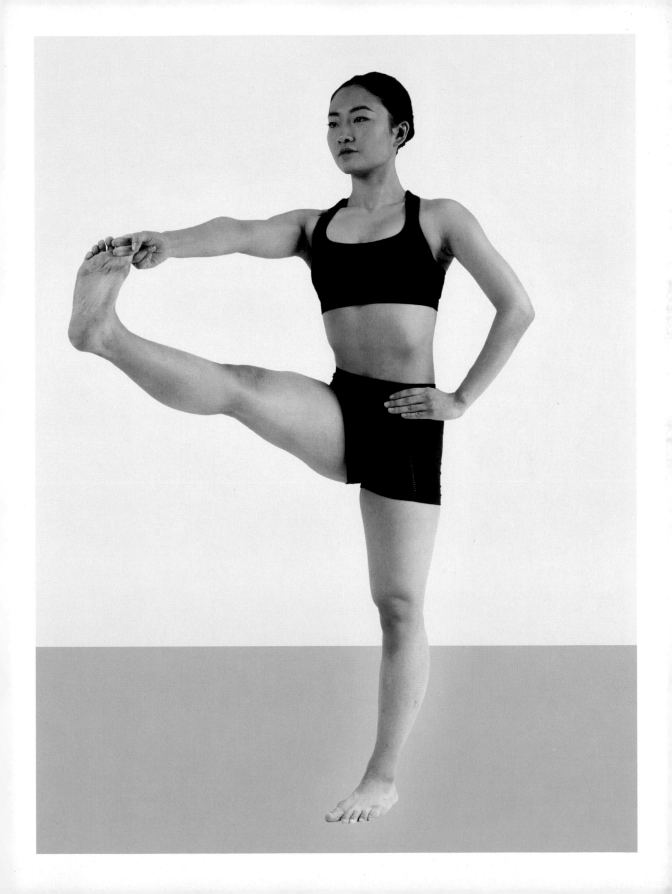

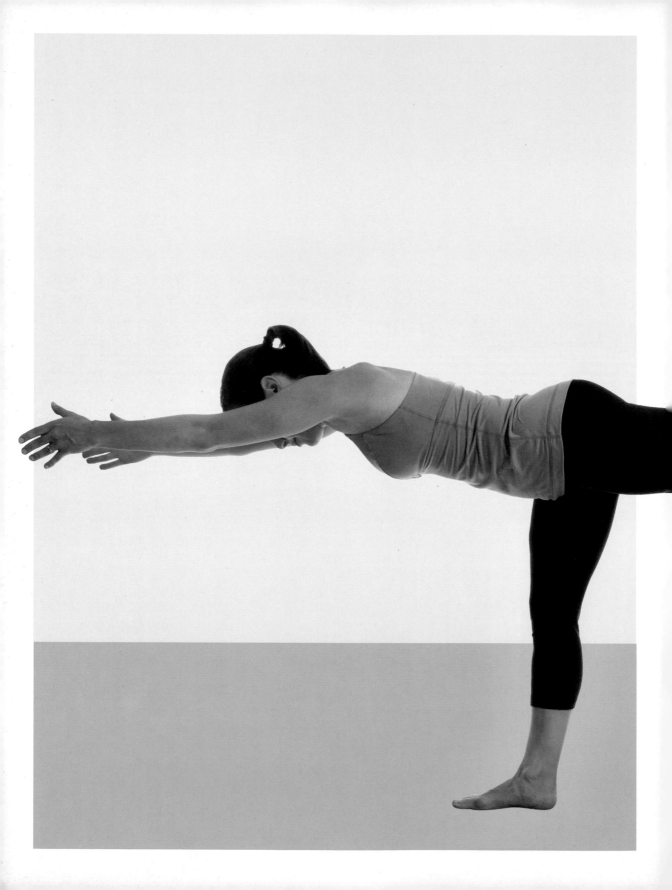

Warrior III Pose

FIND YOUR FORM

Energizing the lifted leg will help you to balance. Keep your hips squared, your neck neutral, and your spine elongated.

Some yoga manuals describe VIRABHADRASANA III as an intermediate pose, others consider it an advanced pose. There is no arguing that it is a demanding asana, one that will effectively work your arms, shoulders, and upper back as well as toning your abdominals. Warrior III is often found in yoga sequences.

BE CAREFUL OF...

Do not let your lifted leg bend or hang without any control. Avoid this pose if you suffer from headaches or low blood pressure.

VARIATIONS

One-Handed Warrior III: For a less difficult pose, extend only one hand and place the other on an upturned yoga block.

Warrior III Squat: Test your balance by trying the pose with the supporting knee bent out over the toes.

STEPS

1. Start in Mountain Pose (p.16) standing in the middle of your mat with your feet together, arms relaxed. Step your right foot about two feet forward.
2. Raise your arms straight overhead, palms facing. Raise your left heel slightly off the ground as you shift your weight to the ball of your forward right foot.
3. With arms still extended, hinge forward over your right thigh, pressing all four corners of your right foot into the mat to ground you.
4. Gradually raise your left leg behind you until it reaches hip height, then flex your foot. Your outstretched arms and raised leg should be parallel to the floor.
5. Hold for two to five breaths before repeating on the other side.

Bowing with Respect Pose

FIND YOUR FORM

Keep your supporting knee positioned over your ankle. Use your extended free arm to maintain your balance.

BE CAREFUL OF...

Avoid this pose if you have shoulder, hip, or knee issues, low blood pressure, or headaches.

For another take on the Warrior III pose, try this advanced pose, which calls for strength, balance, and flexibility. It offers a great stretch to the shoulders, spine, and hamstrings, and strengthens the ankles, thighs, core, and spine while it opens the hips.

STEPS

1. Start out in Warrior III Pose (p.62), balanced on your right leg with your left leg raised behind you and your arms extended in front.
2. Bend your raised leg and bring the knee forward beneath your torso. Reach down and grab your toes with your left hand and extend both arm and leg out to the left side.
3. Spread the toes on your supporting foot to keep you grounded.
4. Hold the pose for two to four breaths before switching sides.

VARIATION

Prop Aid: If you have trouble straightening your raised leg, wrap a yoga strap around the sole of your foot and grasp that as you extend your left arm.

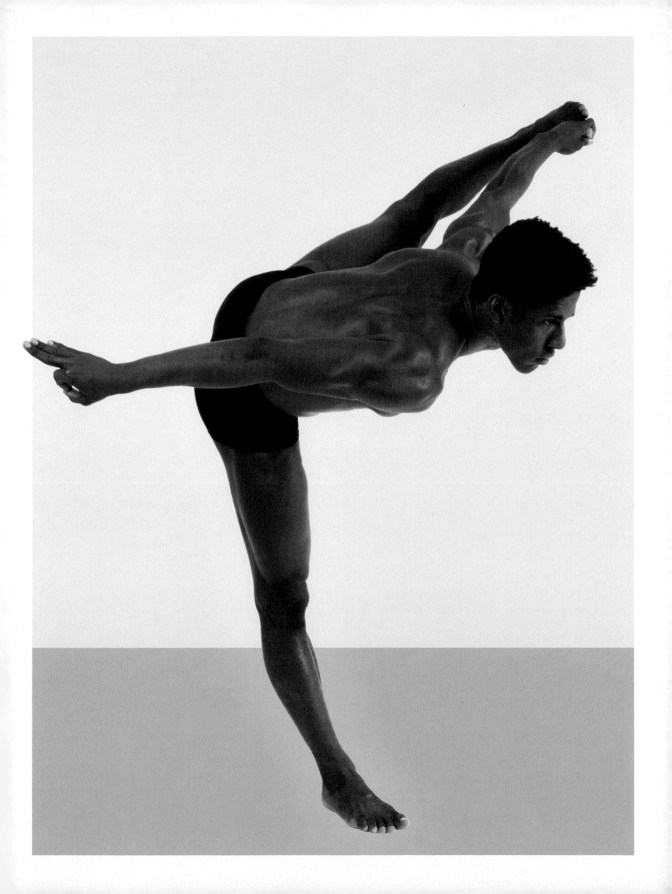

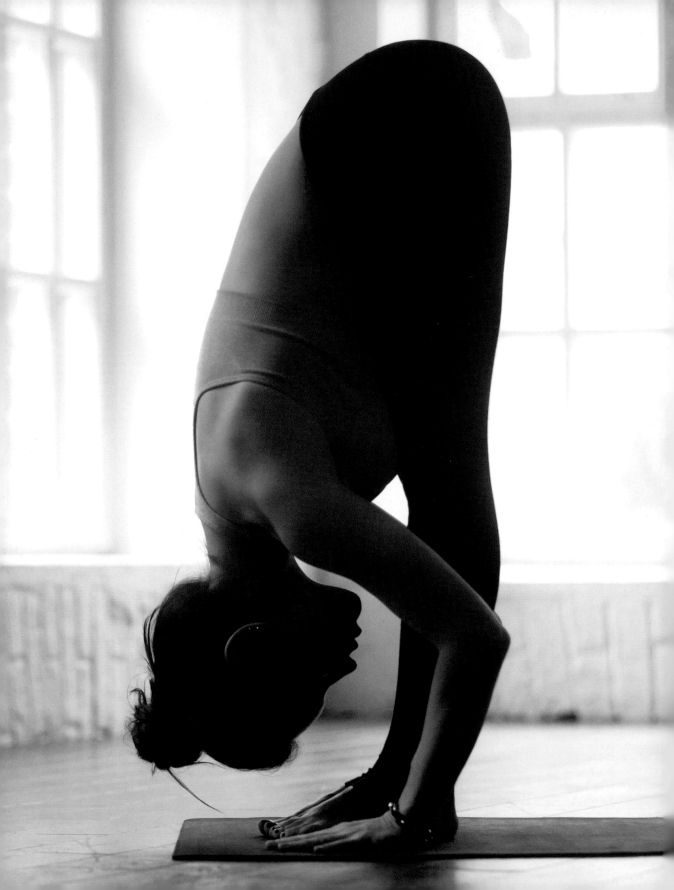

CHAPTER TWO

Standing Forward Bends

These poses are known for stretching the whole body, but especially the spine and the backs of the legs, including the hamstrings. Because they are weight bearing, standing bends work to strengthen the legs and pelvis. They can also help combat stress and ease nervous conditions—as you lower your head downward into each pose, you will feel tension and tightness begin to release.

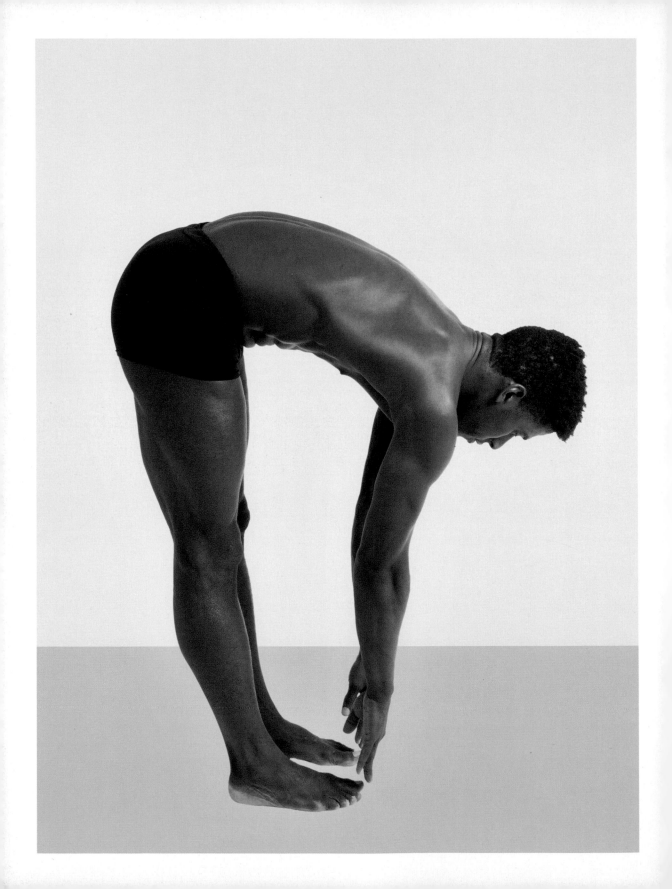

BEGINNER

INTERMEDIATE

ADVANCED

Standing Toe Touch

FIND YOUR FORM

Make sure your knees and thighs are not touching to gain the maximum benefit to your gluteal muscles.

BE CAREFUL OF...

Keep your neck in neutral position as you gaze at the floor. Avoid this pose if you have back issues.

This beginner pose is useful for providing a deep stretch along the spine and the back of the legs before engaging in a sequence of poses. It's helpful for beginner students to understand the point is not to actually touch your toes but to activate your back and legs.

STEPS

1. Stand upright with your arms relaxed, your knees slightly bent, and your feet placed shoulder-width apart.
2. Slowly round your spine from your neck to your lumbar region as you lower your arms toward your feet and reach with outstretched fingers for your toes.
3. Bend at the waist as you continue lowering your torso, letting the weight of your body draw you even farther down. Hold for three to six breaths.

VARIATION

Alternate Toe Touch: Rather than reaching down with both hands, try reaching for the left toes with the right hand, then switch sides. Place the unused hand behind your waist.

INTERMEDIATE

ADVANCED

Standing Half Forward Bend

FIND YOUR FORM

Keep a slight bend in your knees if your hamstrings are tight.

BE CAREFUL OF...

Avoid compressing your neck as you gaze forward.

STEPS

1. Begin in Mountain Pose (p.16), inhale and raise your arms to the ceiling.

2. Hinge forward as you reach down toward your toes with both hands, fingertips straight. Be sure to spread your toes and press down evenly through all four corners of your feet.

3. Keep your back straight except for a slight backbend in your upper back as you broaden your chest and draw in your stomach.

4. Lift your tailbone toward the ceiling as you plant your fingertips in line with your toes and gaze forward. Hold the pose for three to six breaths.

VARIATION

Optional Mode: If your back, neck, or shoulders are stiff, place your hands on your shins rather than reaching for your toes.

This beginner pose acts as a prep for the Standing Forward Bend. Also known as ARDHA UTTANASANA, the Standing Half Forward Bend is a key part of the Sun Salutations and can prepare students for deeper poses. It not only stretches and rejuvenates the spine, calves, hips, and hamstrings, it is ideal for relieving stress.

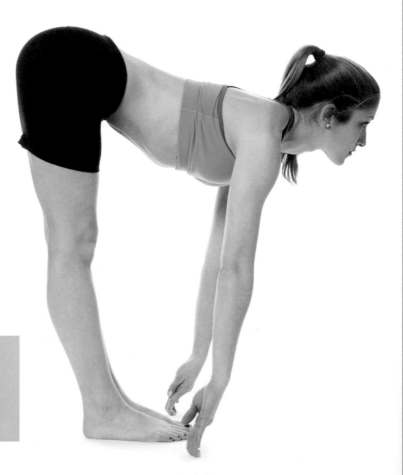

BEGINNER

INTERMEDIATE

ADVANCED

Standing Forward Bend

FIND YOUR FORM

Make sure your hips remain in line with your heels; do not roll your spine into or out of the pose.

BE CAREFUL OF...

Avoid this pose if you have low-back or neck issues or osteoporosis.

STEPS

1. From Standing Half Forward Bend, inhale to lengthen your spine as you begin to transition into Standing Forward Bend.

2. Exhale as you bend forward from the hips while keeping your legs straight, and place your palms on the floor.

3. Lengthen your torso as you bring your belly closer to your thighs. Press your heels to the floor and raise your tailbone to the ceiling. Hold this position as you inhale and exhale three to five times.

VARIATION

Block Aid: Use blocks if you cannot quite flatten your palms on the floor.

Also known as UTTANASANA, the Standing Forward Bend is often used in sequences and combinations. It stretches the hamstrings, hips, and spine while strengthening the thighs and knees. By performing both Half Forward and Forward Bend repeatedly, you will soon be able to deepen your fold into the final bend.

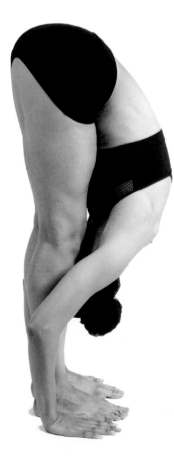

BEGINNER
INTERMEDIATE
ADVANCED

Side Bend to Half Forward Bend Circle

FIND YOUR FORM

Make sure to keep your arms straight and your hips above your feet, not behind them.

BE CAREFUL OF...

Students who suffer from lower-back issues should avoid this pose.

This versatile pose is useful for toning the core and shoulder muscles as well as those of the upper body. It also stretches the spine and obliques and can help correct poor posture while it improves overall flexibility.

STEPS

1. Begin in Mountain Pose (p.16) with your arms relaxed and your feet together.
2. Raise both arms over your head and lace your fingers together, with your palms facing up.
3. While keeping your elbows straight, reach out with your arms to the left side.
4. Using your torso, begin tracing a circle pattern with your arms.
5. Lean forward and then to the right as you continue to create the circle shape.
6. End with your arms again over your head. Repeat three times, then return to Mountain Pose, and circle in the opposite direction.

VARIATION

The Sweep: While creating the front part of the circle, trying sweeping your arms down toward the floor.

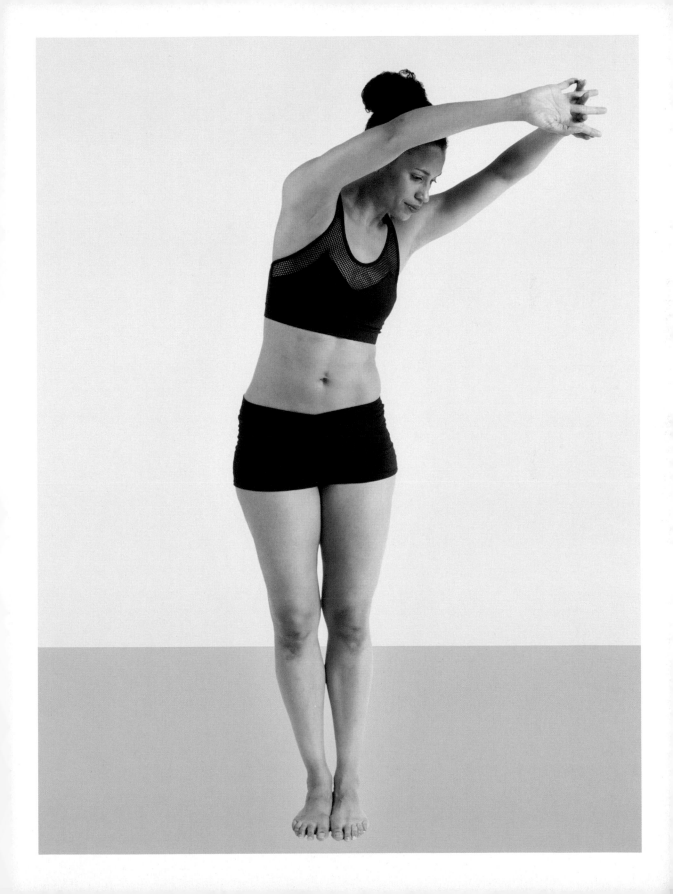

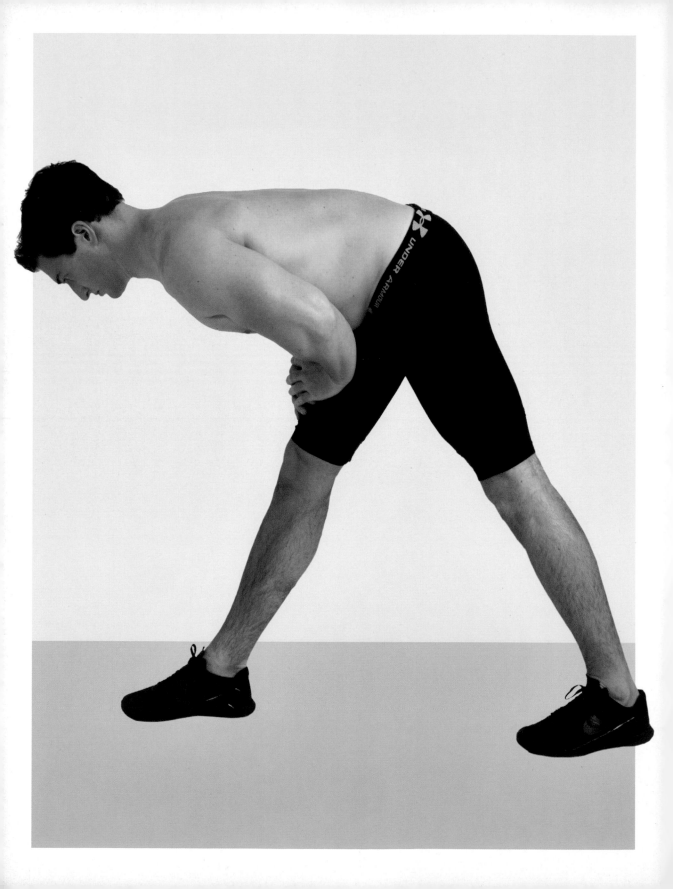

Straight-Leg Lunge Pose

This beginner pose provides a great stretch for the lower back, hamstrings, and calves. It also works to improve mid- and lower-body balance by strengthening the core, legs, and buttocks. Try practicing this pose if you have issues with hip mobility or spinal pain flare-ups.

FIND YOUR FORM

Keep your chest elevated and your torso elongated. To maximize the stretch, flex your forward foot by lifting the ball of the foot off the floor.

BE CAREFUL OF...

Try not to retain unnecessary tension in your upper body. If you have neck issues, it is best to avoid this pose.

STEPS

1. Stand upright with your arms relaxed and your feet parallel and shoulder-width apart.
2. Bend your knees slightly as you tip your pelvis forward. Elevate your chest, and press your shoulders down and back.
3. Take a long step forward with your right leg and then lean your torso forward over your extended knee. Place both hands on your right knee to help you maintain your balance. Keep both legs straight.
4. As you lean forward, the weight of your body will intensify the stretch. Be sure to keep your rear heel on the floor and your gaze on your forward foot.
5. Hold for three to six breaths before standing and repeating on the left side.

VARIATION

Hands Down: From the completed Lunge Pose, stretch your hands down, and place your palms on the floor.

BEGINNER
INTERMEDIATE
ADVANCED

Intense Side Stretch Pose

This intermediate pose, also called PARSVOTTANASANA, stretches the legs, shoulders, spine, and wrists. It helps to strengthen the legs and spine, while improving poor posture and de-stressing both mind and body.

FIND YOUR FORM

Make sure not to round your back as you bend forward. For tight hamstrings, try widening your stance.

BE CAREFUL OF...

Avoid this pose if you suffer from hamstring or spine problems.

STEPS

1. Begin in Mountain Pose (p.16), then step your left leg back two or three feet.
2. Angle your toes toward the left front corner of the mat and bring them into heel-to-heel alignment while keeping your hips squared to the front of the mat.
3. Bring your hands behind your back, and place them palm to palm, fingers down. Rotate your hand inward to reverse prayer position, finger pointing up.
4. Inhale to increase the space across your collarbone and lift your chest.
5. Ground yourself with the pinky of your rear foot, and press your rear thigh back as you exhale and lean forward over your right leg, bringing your chest close to your thigh.
6. Keeping your spine elongated and your gaze on the ground, hold the pose for three to six breaths. Inhale, draw your shoulders back, raise your sternum, and return to standing position. Repeat on the other side.

VARIATION

Deep Bend: From the completed pose, fold your body down as close to your forward thigh as possible with your crown facing the floor.

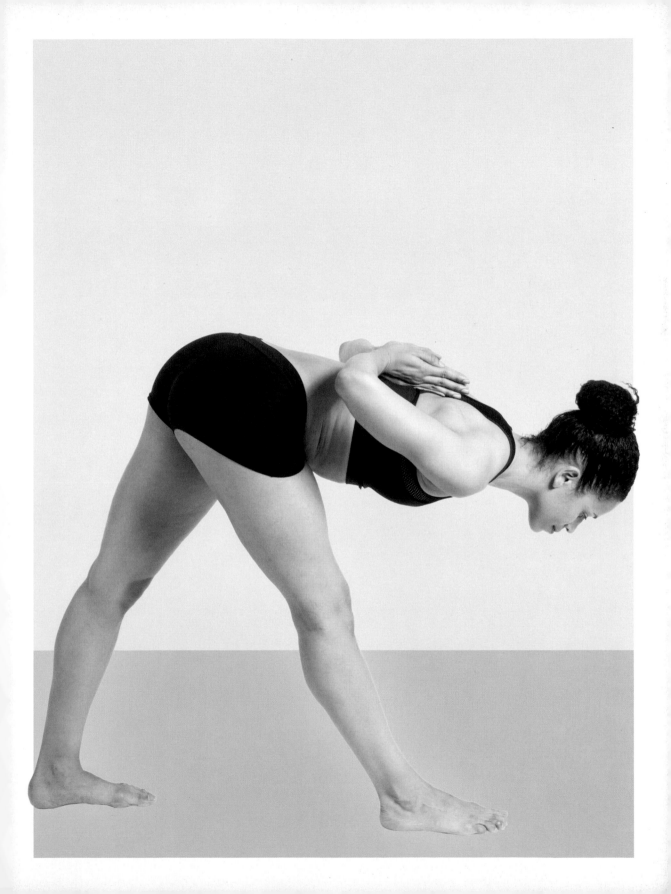

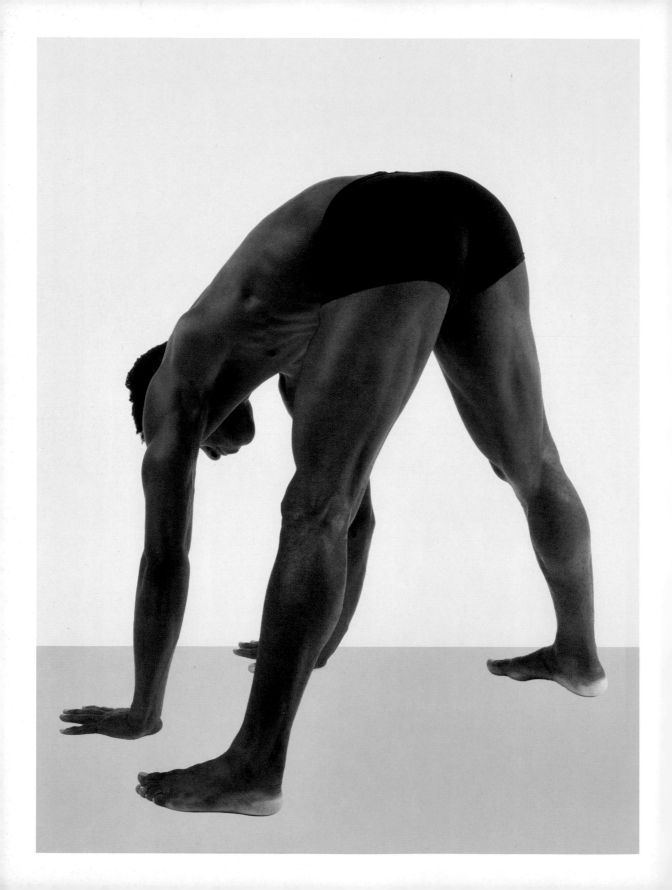

BEGINNER
INTERMEDIATE
ADVANCED

Wide-Legged Forward Bend

FIND YOUR FORM
Bend only as far as is comfortable with your back flat. Keep your hips aligned with your heels, not behind them.

BE CAREFUL OF...
Avoid locking your knees as you reach down; keep them as soft as possible.

Also known as PRASARITA PADOTTANASANA, this intermediate pose offers a deep stretch to the back, hips, and hamstrings while it opens the groin. It is a favorite pose of dancers, who often use it to calm their nerves before a performance.

STEPS
1. Begin by standing upright with your feet more than shoulder-width apart and your knees slightly bent. Tuck your pelvis forward, and draw your shoulder blades in.
2. Lengthen your spine as you inhale, lift your chest, and create a small bend in your upper back as you raise your gaze to the ceiling.
3. Keeping your back flat, hinge forward from the waist on an exhale, and place your palms flat on the floor in front of you. Bring your crown toward the floor as you bring your shoulders toward your ears.
4. Firm up your thighs, and lift your kneecaps. Raise your sit bones toward the ceiling as your tailbone angles toward the floor. Hold for four to six breaths.

VARIATIONS
Block Aid: If you cannot reach the floor at first, use yoga blocks.
Head Rest: For a challenge, walk your hands back between your legs, bend your elbows, and rest your forehead on the floor.

BEGINNER
INTERMEDIATE
ADVANCED

Crossed-Foot Forward Bend

FIND YOUR FORM

Make sure to keep your knees straight but not locked during the pose.

BE CAREFUL OF...

Try not to twist your neck or shoulders as you bend. Avoid this pose if you have hip injuries.

This forward bend works great for improving flexibility as it stretches the hamstrings, upper and lower back, and calves. The crossed-foot position also targets the iliotibial band, the fibrous tissue that runs along the outer thigh, as well as stabilizing your hip and knee joints. This pose also helps to counteract the effects of wearing high-heeled shoes.

STEPS

1. Stand upright with your arms relaxed at your sides.
2. Cross one foot over the other until the outer sides of your soles are aligned.
3. Bend forward from the waist and gradually reach down toward the floor.
4. With your body folded close to your thighs, let your head drop, and press your palms to the floor. Hold for three to five breaths.
5. Gently roll up into standing position, and repeat the pose with the opposite feet crossed.

VARIATION

Optional Mode: If you find it difficult at first to touch the floor, reach down as far as is comfortable. Then extend your reach a bit each time you practice this pose.

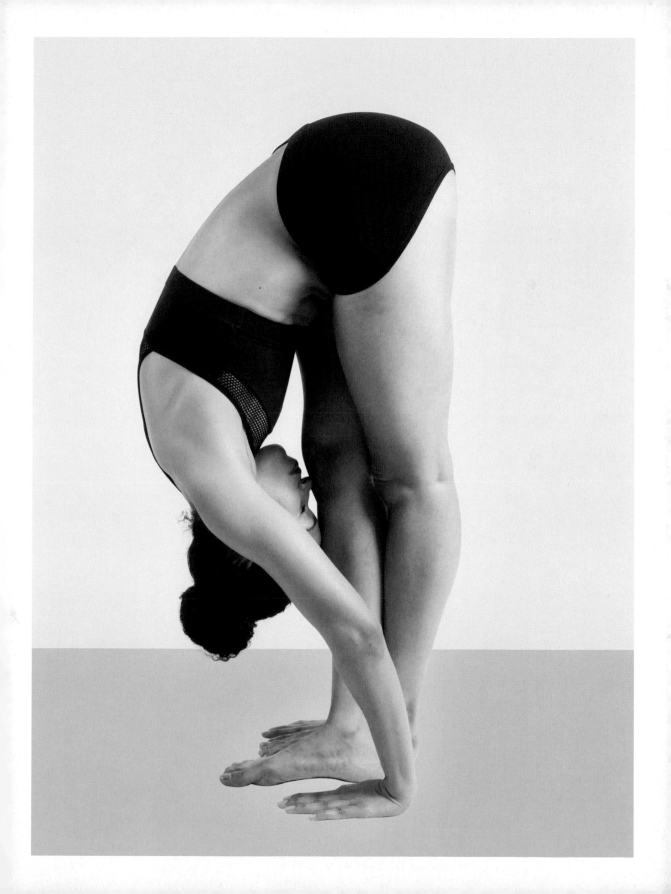

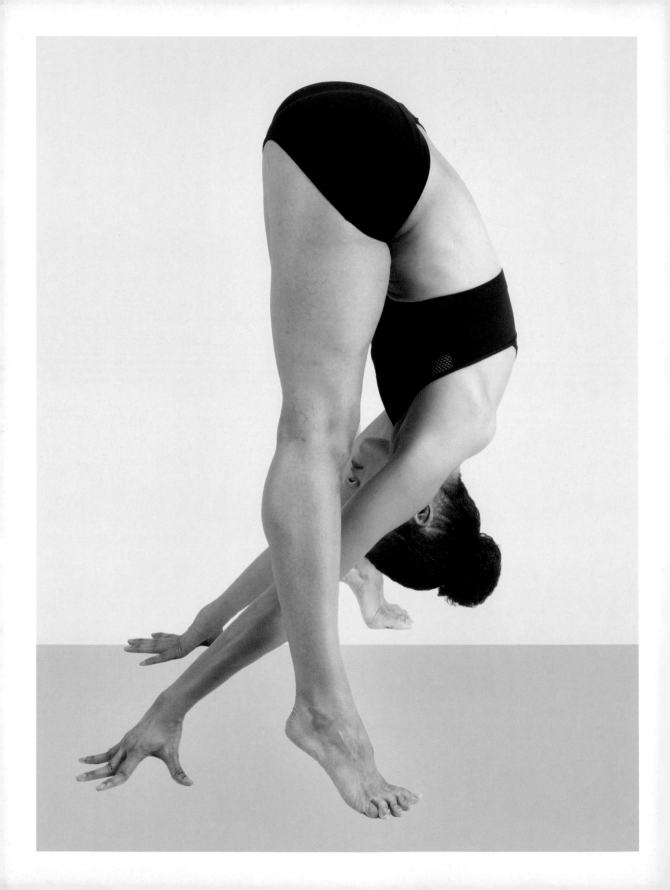

BEGINNER

INTERMEDIATE

ADVANCED

Tiptoe Intense Stretch Pose

FIND YOUR FORM

Create a stable platform to balance on using your legs and your outstretched fingers. Concentrate on bringing your torso as close to your thighs as possible.

BE CAREFUL OF...

Try to eliminate any tension in your neck. Avoid this pose if you suffer from wrist or ankle pain or have balance issues.

This advanced pose, known as PRAPADA UTTANASANA in Sanskrit, stretches the spine, abdominals, and glutes while easing tight hamstrings. It is also effective for improving your sense of balance. The pose can be considered an inversion since you heart ends up higher than your head.

STEPS

1. Start by standing in Half Forward Bend Pose (p.70), then shift your feet to shoulder-width apart.
2. Raise yourself up on tiptoes, and reach back between your legs; Spread your arms and touch the floor with your fingertips. Round the middle of your back as you straighten your arms, and lower your head to gaze back through your legs at your hands.
3. Hold for three to six breaths.

VARIATION

Tiptoe Half Intense Stretch: For less of a challenge, when folding down, reach only for the floor in front of you with your fingertips rather than reaching between your legs.

Standing Split Pose Prep

FIND YOUR FORM

Firm up your leg muscles as you ground your standing foot into the mat. Keep your back and legs straight.

BE CAREFUL OF...

Do not compress the back of your neck while holding the pose. Avoid this asana if you suffer from ankle or knee issues or have lower-back pain.

This advanced pose, called URDHVA PRASARITA EKA PADASANA, is both a forward bend and an inversion. Standing splits are often a part of dance training, but don't be intimidated—this is an excellent pose for stretching your lower body and legs while prepping for more difficult split poses.

STEPS

1. Start in Mountain Pose (p.16), and lift your arms overhead, shoulder-width apart.
2. Hinge forward from the hips; as you bring your weight forward, reach down with both hands and press your fingertips to the floor about a foot in front of your toes.
3. Keeping your hips squared, shift your weight onto your left leg, and raise your right leg until it is in line with your back. Flex your right foot, toes down.
4. Hold the pose for three to five breaths before switching sides.

VARIATIONS

Prop Aid: If you have trouble touching the ground, place your hands on two yoga blocks.

Ankle Grab: For a balance challenge, grasp the ankle of your standing leg with both hands as you externally rotate the hip of your raised leg.

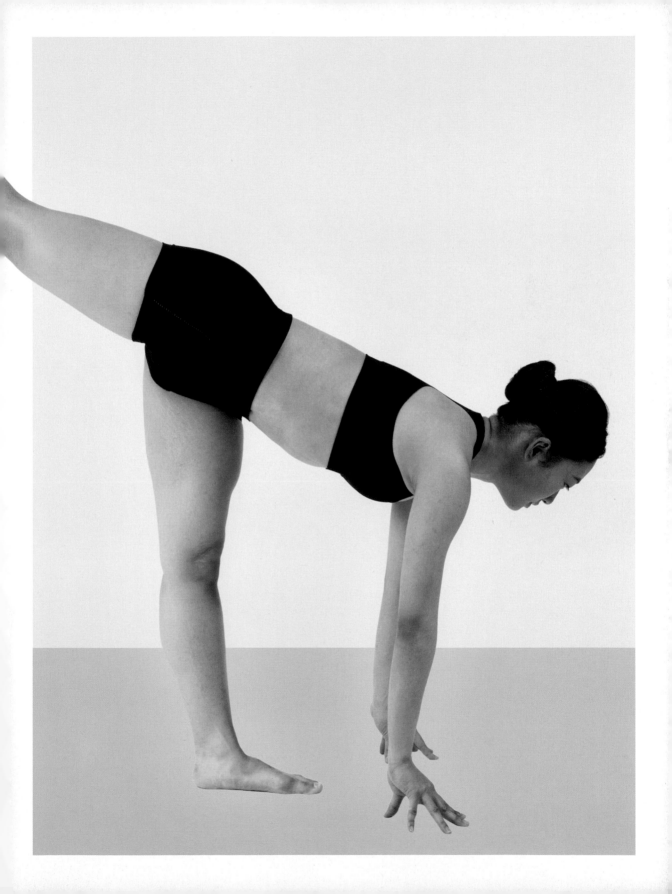

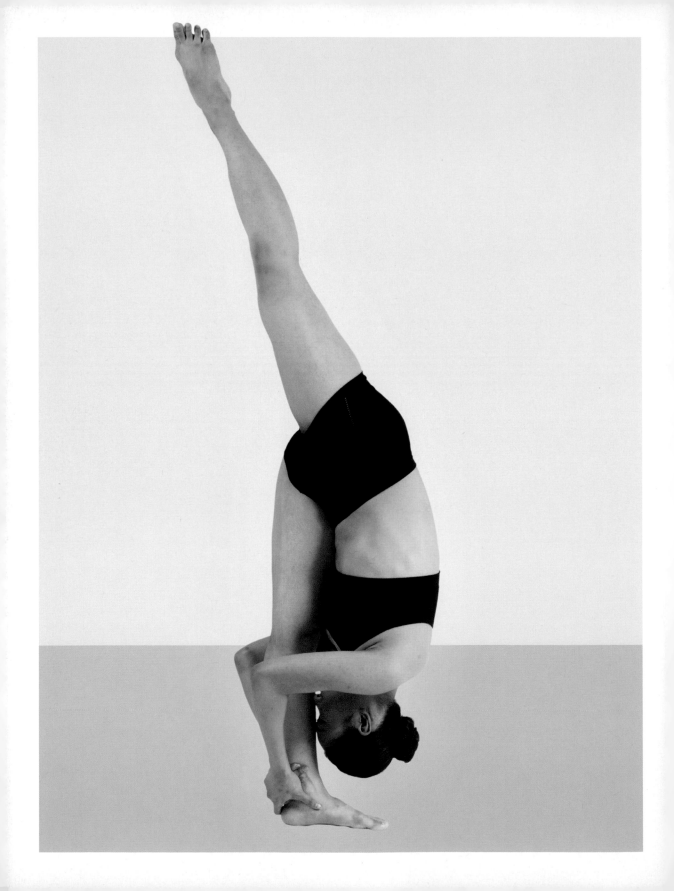

BEGINNER
INTERMEDIATE
ADVANCED

Standing Split Pose

FIND YOUR FORM

Elongate the back of your neck as you tuck your chin into your chest.

BE CAREFUL OF...

Do not allow your supporting knee to rotate inward. Avoid this pose if you suffer from wrist or ankle pain or have balance issues.

This advanced pose should be worked up to gradually and only performed when you are warmed up. Once you have mastered it, you will benefit from deep stretching of the groin, thighs, and calves, and strengthening of the thighs, knees, and ankles. Your sense of balance will also be noticeably improved.

STEPS

1. Begin standing in Mountain Pose (p.16), and then shift your weight onto your left foot.
2. Bend forward from your hips, place your fingertips on the floor in front of you and raise your right leg behind you.
3. On an exhale, tighten your leg muscles, and ease your torso down as close to your left thigh as you can manage. At the same time, raise your right leg toward the ceiling, toes flexed or pointed.
4. Try to grasp the back of your left ankle with both hands. Or place your left palm on the floor to help you balance.
5. Hold for three to five breaths before switching sides.

VARIATION

Tripod Split: For a less challenging version of this pose, after Step 3, stretch your outspread arms on the floor in front of you, palms down.

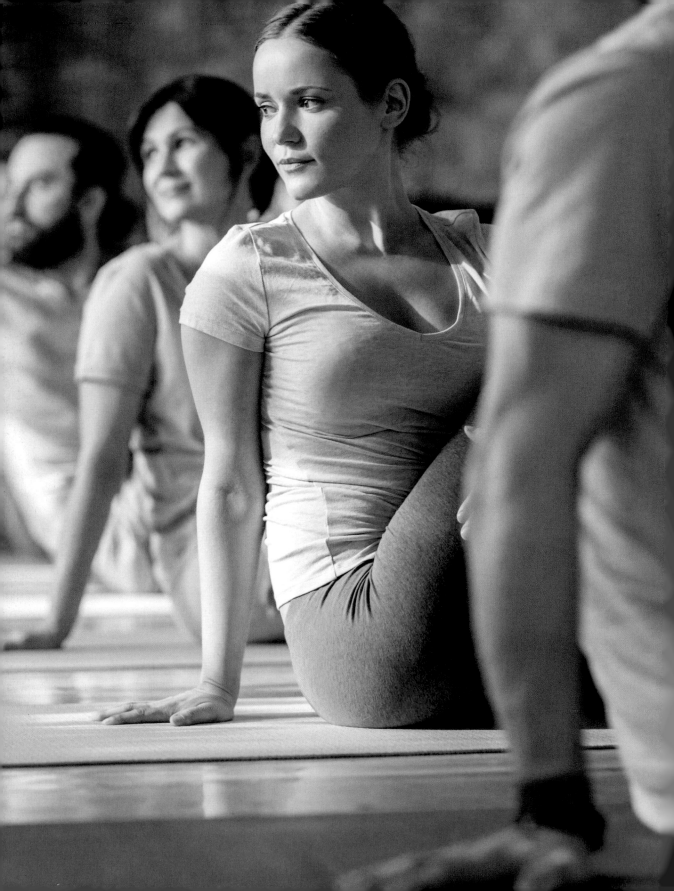

CHAPTER THREE

Seated Poses and Twists

Perhaps the best thing about seated poses and twists is that they are accessible to most beginners—students get to work on flexibility, build strength, and improve breathing techniques while in a position of stability. Seated asanas can especially help tone the abdominal muscles, the obliques, the lower back, and the upper thighs. They also offer mental and spiritual benefits such as clarity, calmness, insight, and increased confidence.

BEGINNER

BEGINNER

INTERMEDIATE

ADVANCED

Easy Pose

SUKHASANA, a basic, cross-legged beginner pose, stems from the hatha tradition and is often used during meditation. This asana may look uncomplicated, but performing it correctly can be challenging if your muscles are stiff. It strengthens the back and abdominals and stretches the knees and ankles while opening the groin and hips.

FIND YOUR FORM

Make sure you do not allow your knees to rise above the level of your hips; keep your shoulders squared.

BE CAREFUL OF...

Do not attempt this pose if you have severe leg problems.

STEPS

1. Sit on the floor with your knees bent and your legs crossed at the shins. The outer edge of each foot should be on the mat.
2. Press your sit bones down to the floor to create a neutral pelvis.
3. Elongate your spine and open your collarbones as you draw your torso upright.
4. Place your hands on your thighs, either palm down or palm up.
5. Close your eyes and focus on your breathing, increasing the length of inhalation and exhalation, eventually making them of the same duration. Hold for six to ten breaths, or as long as is comfortable before switching legs.

VARIATION

Prop Aid: If this pose is difficult at first, try sitting on a yoga block or folded blanket to elevate your hips.

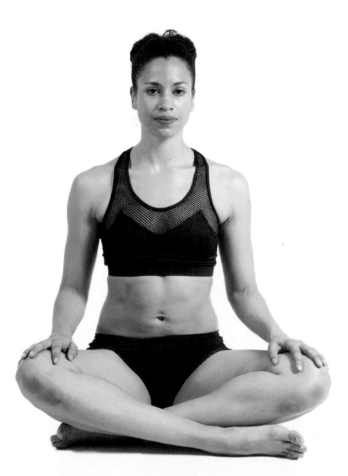

Staff Pose

FIND YOUR FORM

Keep your pelvis in neutral position, and draw your shoulder blades together.

BE CAREFUL OF...

Make sure you don't stick out your ribs while in hold. Avoid this pose if you have tight hamstrings or lower-back pain.

STEPS

1. Begin by sitting on the mat with your legs together and outstretched in front of you. Activate your legs by firming your thighs to the floor, flexing your feet, and pressing your heels forward.
2. Put your weight on the front of your sit bones as you root your tailbone to the floor. Place your arms at your sides with your palms on the floor.
3. Use your abdominal muscles to help your energy rise upward from your tailbone to your crown.
4. Hold the pose for six to ten breaths, or for however long is comfortable.

Also known as DANDASANA, Staff Pose is the foundational asana for many other seated poses. It may appear simple at first, but in order to enjoy the stretching and strengthening benefits to the legs and spine, it needs to be performed perfectly.

VARIATION

Prop Aid: If you find your pelvis keeps tucking under or your lower back is rounding when you straighten your legs, sit on a yoga block or folded blanket.

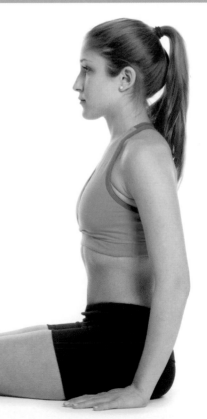

Bound Angle Pose

FIND YOUR FORM

Be sure you are sitting up tall; aim for a straight line from your sit bones to your shoulders.

BE CAREFUL OF...

If you experience thigh or groin pain, sit on a folded blanket. This pose should be avoided if you suffer from knee or groin injuries.

Bound Angle Pose, or BADDHA KONASANA, is also known as the Tailor Pose because tailors in India often sit in this fashion to work. This beginner pose stretches the inner thighs, groin, and knees and can help relieve the pain of menstrual cramps.

STEPS

1. Bend your knees and lower them outward; bring your soles together as you draw your feet in toward your pelvis.
2. Hold your feet together and press the pinky sides of your feet to ground, opening the upper sole like a book.
3. While keeping your spine neutral, draw your lower torso upward, and spread your weight equally over your sit bones.
4. Hold for six to nine breaths.

VARIATIONS

Prayer Hands: While sitting in Bound Angle Pose, draw your torso upward and press the soles of your feet together as you form prayer hands at your chest.

Bending Forward: From Bound Angle Pose, elongate your torso and spine and lean forward until your chest is over your feet. Hold for five to 10 breaths.

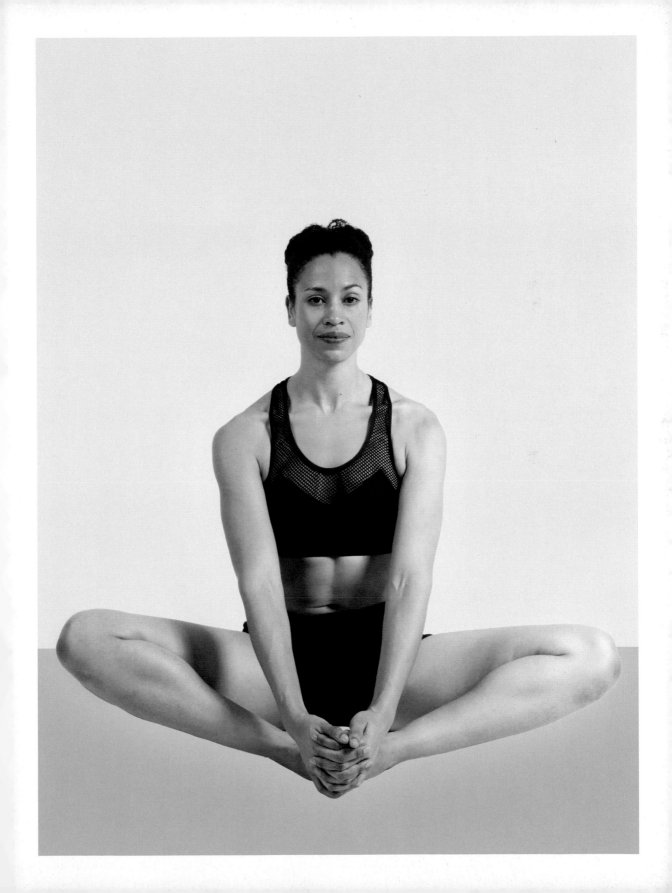

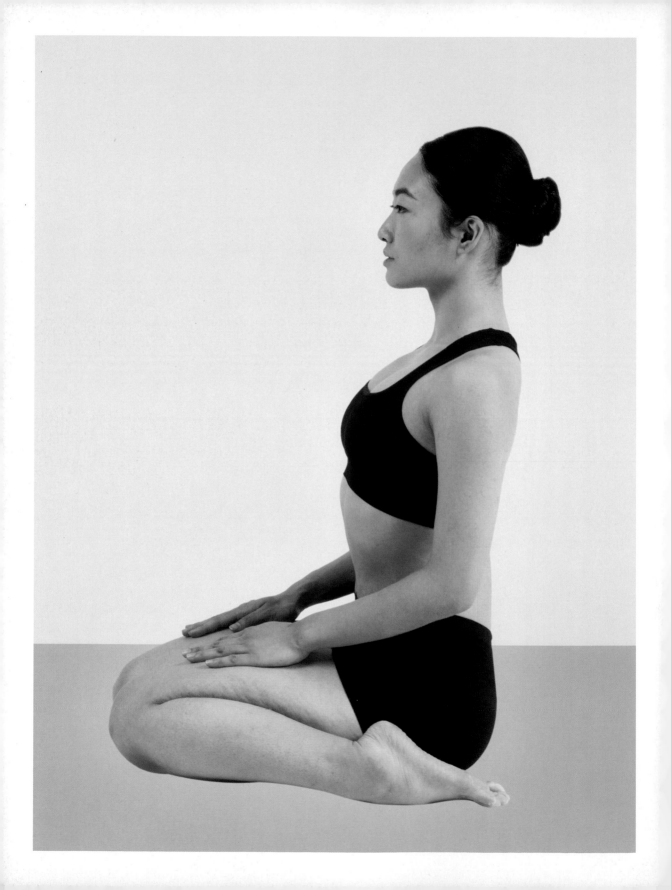

Hero Pose

FIND YOUR FORM

To help make room for your buttocks between your legs, place your thumbs behind your knees and gently roll the flesh of the calves outward.

BE CAREFUL OF...

While in pose, don't let your ribs jut forward or your back hollow out. Avoid this pose if you have knee or ankle issues.

VIRASANA strengthens the arches of the foot while stretching the thighs, knees, and ankles. It is therapeutic for tired legs after a long day on your feet. This pose traces back to medieval hatha yoga, which described it as a meditation asana, and it does make a less-challenging alternative to Lotus Pose for that purpose.

STEPS

1. Kneel on the mat with your legs hip-width apart, thighs perpendicular to the floor, and soles facing up.
2. Bring your knees together, and move your heels to slightly wider than hip-width apart.
3. Lower your buttocks down between your heels as you keep your torso upright. Internally rotate your thighs, and lengthen your tailbone between your heels as you raise your public bone upward.
4. Place your palms on your thighs—facing upward to receive energy or downward for a calming effect. Hold for four to six breaths.

VARIATIONS

Supported Hero: To aid tight knees, kneel on a fold blanket or towel so that your ankles jut off the blanket's edge. Place a yoga block between your spread heels before easing back and sitting up.

Deep Stretch Hero: To increase the stretch, place your forearms on the mat behind you, and lean back on your elbows.

BEGINNER

INTERMEDIATE

ADVANCED

Cat Pose

FIND YOUR FORM

Breathe space between your shoulder blades, and be sure to keep your shoulders over your wrists as your back arches.

BE CAREFUL OF...

Don't force your chin into your chest. If you have neck pain, keep your head aligned with your body; avoid the pose if you have wrist issues.

STEPS

1. Start down on all fours in "tabletop" position, with your hands placed below your shoulders, fingers spread, knees below your hips, and toes facing back. Your hips should be in neutral position.
2. Ground your hands down into the mat with your thumbs and forefingers as you rotate your arms externally, away from your center line.
3. Lower your head, and begin to round your upper back as you draw your abdomen in toward your spine. Keep your shoulders and knees in correct alignment as you arch up.
4. Gaze back toward your navel as you hold the pose for four to eight breaths before exhaling and returning to tabletop position.

This kneeling beginner pose, also known as MARJARYASANA, can greatly increase flexibility in the spine, especially when the student moves one vertebra at a time, a process called articulation. Cat Pose stretches the upper body while it strengthens the wrists and hands.

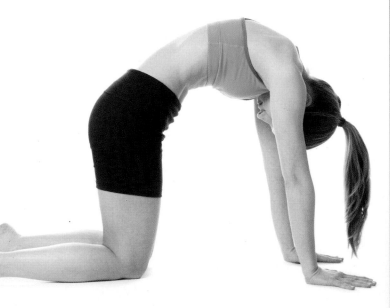

VARIATION
Raise Up: To activate your core during the pose, briefly lift your knees and your wrists from the mat just enough distance to slide a paper beneath them.

Cow Pose

FIND YOUR FORM
To keep your lower back from drooping, draw your stomach muscles inward toward your spine.

BE CAREFUL OF...
Avoid this pose if you have neck or wrist issues.

This beginner pose, also known as BITILASANA or Dog Tilt Pose, provides a mild backbend, furnishing the student with a gentle preparation for more demanding backbends. Cow Pose is frequently performed in tandem with Cat Pose as a warm-up sequence to increase flexibility in the spine.

STEPS
1. Start down on all fours in "tabletop" position, with your hands placed below your shoulders, fingers spread, knees below your hips, and toes facing back. Your hips should be in neutral position.
2. Press down through your knuckles to ground yourself.
3. Inhale, then raise your sternum and your sit bones as you create a hollow in the middle of your back.
4. Tilt your head back, and lift your gaze to the center of your forehead (or third eye). Hold the pose for four to eight breaths before returning to tabletop position.

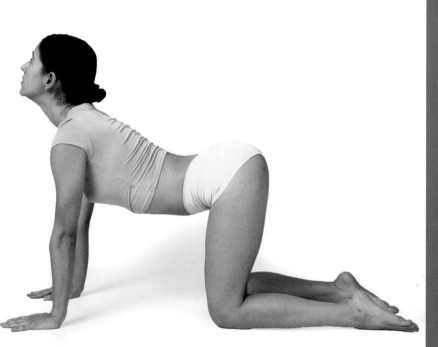

VARIATION
Breath Retention: During the Cat/Cow sequence, try holding an inhale of five seconds during Cow Pose and holding a similar exhale during Cat Pose.

BEGINNER

INTERMEDIATE

ADVANCED

Marichi's Pose

FIND YOUR FORM

Position both sit bones on the floor and keep your shoulders relaxed. Use your upper torso to twist your spine more completely.

BE CAREFUL OF...

Try not to hunch your shoulders up to your ears or round your spine. Never force your spine into a twist. Avoid this pose if you have back or knee issues or suffer from high or low blood pressure.

VARIATIONS

Marichi Prep: You can work up to the final pose by sitting on a block or folded blanket and raising your rear arm, palm flat, to a wall for support.

Tiptoe Half Strap Option: To increase the stretch, from this final pose place a yoga strap around the instep of your outstretched foot, and hold it taut with both hands while maintaining the twist in your torso.

The full name of this asana, Pose Dedicated to the Sage Marichi III (MARICHYASANA III), honors the Hindu seer who intuited the divine law of the universe. A beginner twist, it both stretches and strengthens the spine, opens the hips, stimulates digestion, and removes toxins from the body.

STEPS

1. Begin in Staff Pose (p.91) with legs extended, and bend your left knee as you draw your heel toward your groin. Inhale as you lift up through your spine and concentrate on grounding your right leg and left foot into the floor; keep your left knee facing up.
2. Exhale and gently rotate—in sequence from your lower spine, toros, and chest—toward your left knee.
3. Press your left fingertips to the floor behind your left hip as your right hand draws your left thigh closer to your abdominals.
4. Hook your right elbow over the outside of your left knee, hand up, palm facing in; lean back slightly, and let your gaze follow the line of your left shoulder.
5. Hold for three to six breaths before switching to the opposite side.

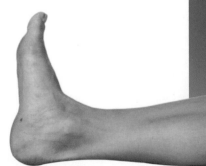

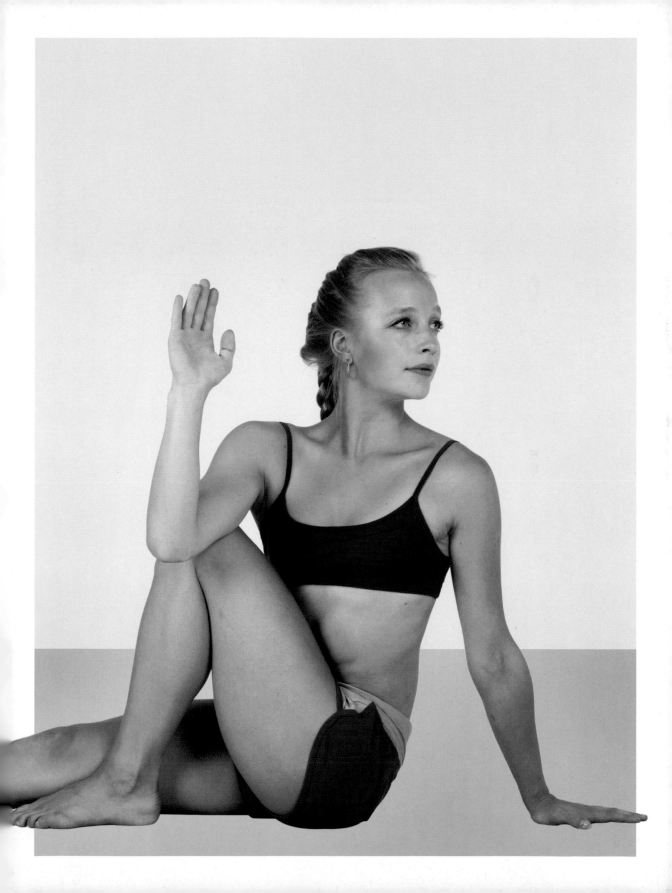

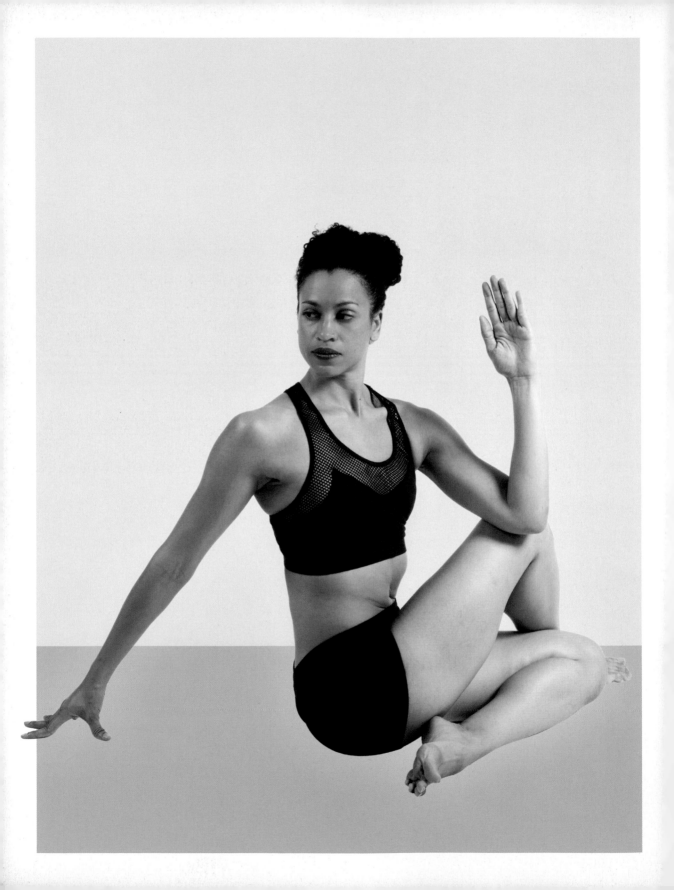

BEGINNER
INTERMEDIATE
ADVANCED

Half Lord of The Fishes Pose

FIND YOUR FORM

Make sure you lengthen your spine as you twist. Draw your shoulder blades together as you widen your collarbones.

BE CAREFUL OF...

Do not twist your neck into any position that causes pain. Avoid this pose if you have spinal issues.

This intermediate seated spinal twist, known as ARDHA MATSYENDRASANA in Sanskrit, provides a deeper stretch than Marichi's Pose. It especially targets the upper body and is useful for stretching the neck, spine, shoulders, and hips. Consider its merits as a long-time cure for digestive issues.

STEPS

1. Begin in Staff Pose (p.91) with your legs extended.
2. Bend your right knee, cross your foot over your left knee, and place it on the outside of your left thigh. Your sole should be flat on the floor. Keep the left knee pointing up.
3. Position your right heel close to your left hip
4. Slide your right arm a foot or more behind your right hip, fingers extended; inhale to create length along your left side as you raise your left arm.
5. On an exhale, ground yourself with both sit bones as you twist your body to the right, and hook your left elbow on the outside of your right thigh. Raise your left hand, palm facing right.
6. Either continue gazing forward or shift your gaze over your right shoulder. Hold for three to six breaths before switching sides.

VARIATIONS

Prop Aid: If you feel your hips are uneven, sit on a block or folded blanket.

Back Handclasp: For a true challenge, work your left forearm back beneath your raised right knee, reach around your back with your right arm, and try to get your hands to meet.

BEGINNER

INTERMEDIATE

ADVANCED

Cow Face Pose

FIND YOUR FORM

While holding the pose, your left elbow should be pointing to the ceiling. Your heels should be an equal distance from your hips.

BE CAREFUL OF...

Do not ask someone to help you link your hands behind your back; this can injure your shoulder or rotator cuff. Avoid this pose if you have shoulder issues or knee problems.

This intermediate pose is also known as GOMUKHASANA in Sanskrit. The crossed knees of the completed pose actually do resemble the lips of a bovine face. It is best to approach the pose by focusing on correct leg alignment before tackling the more demanding arm and hand positions.

STEPS

1. Begin in Staff Pose (p.91), sitting upright with your legs outstretched. Cross your legs at the knees, right over left, and slide your left ankle to the right and your right ankle to the left. Your knees should now be stacked on top of each other.
2. Lift your torso through the spine as you distribute your weight evenly over your sit bones.
3. Inhale, and reach your left hand out to the side. Bend the elbow, and rotate your shoulder down as you reach behind your back. Keep reaching until your hand is between your shoulder blades, palm facing out.
4. On an inhalation, raise your right arm, and reach up toward the ceiling, palm facing behind you. On an exhalation, bend that arm, and reach your left hand down toward the center of your spine.
5. Hook the fingers of both hands together as you raise your chest, and draw your stomach muscles in toward your spine.
6. Keep your gaze forward; hold the pose for three to six breaths before changing sides.

VARIATIONS

Prop Aid: If your two hands can't touch behind your back, grasp a yoga strap or narrow towel to connect them.

Forward Bend: For even more challenge, elongate your spine, lift your raised elbow, and fold forward over your thighs.

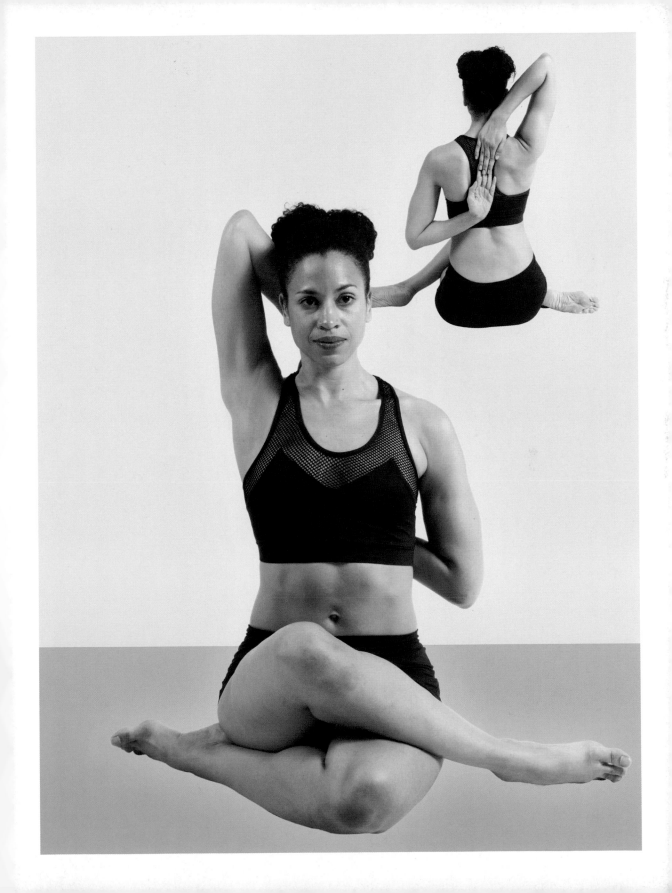

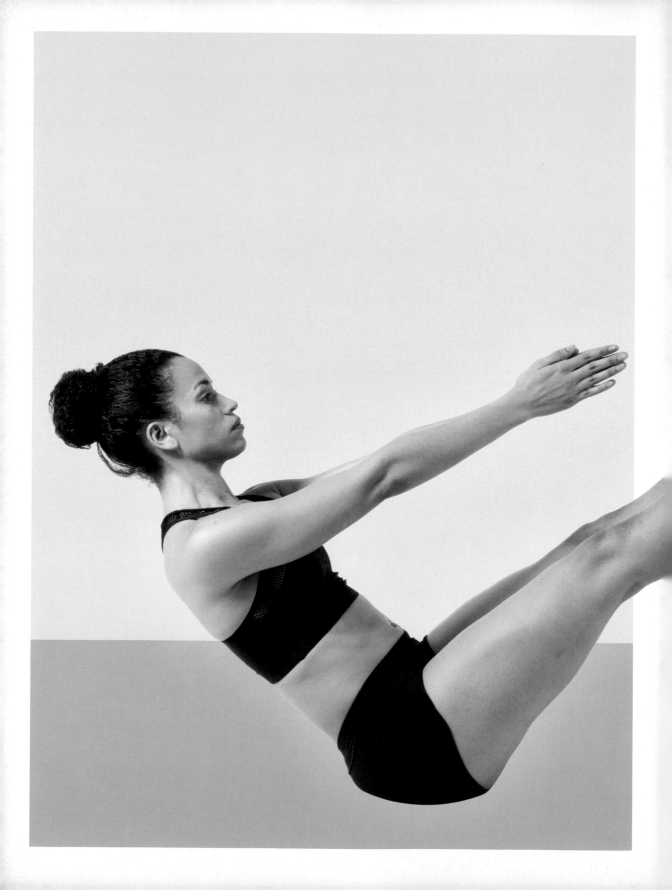

Boat Pose

Boat Pose, or PARIPURNA NAVASANA, is a terrific intermediate pose for building up the muscles of your core and improving stability, in effect grounding your midline while activating it. Plus, the more you practice the pose, the deeper its effects on your stomach, back, and hip flexors.

STEPS

1. Begin in Staff Pose (p.91) with your legs extended.
2. Bend your knees, with your feet flat on the floor, and grasp the outside of your thighs with both hands. Tilt back until you are balanced on your tailbone and two sits bones with your back in a straight line.
3. Raise your legs off the floor until your shins are parallel to the mat. Then extend your arms with the palms facing inward until they are parallel to the floor.
4. On an inhale, gradually straighten your legs so that they create a 45 degree angle from the floor. Your toes should be a bit higher than your head.
5. Internally rotate your thighs to increase stability as you reach forward with fingers and toes and raise your sternum.
6. Tighten your stomach muscles, navel toward spine, as you hold for two to five breaths.

VARIATION

Bent-Knee Version: At first you may find it less taxing to hold the pose at Step 3, with your shins parallel to the floor and your arms outstretched.

FIND YOUR FORM

Be sure to keep your collarbones spaced apart and your legs active.

BE CAREFUL OF...

Do not allow your legs to lower or your stomach to bulge during hold. Avoid this pose if you are pregnant or have a groin injury.

BEGINNER
INTERMEDIATE
ADVANCED

Revolved Supported Boat Pose

FIND YOUR FORM

Elongate your spine as you twist to the side and also concentrate on keeping both legs straight.

BE CAREFUL OF...

Do not over-rotate your head; your face should line up with your left (rear) shoulder. Avoid this pose if you are pregnant or suffer from neck or groin issues.

Also called PARIVRTTA SALAMBA NAVASANA, this is another pose that effectively tones the deeper core muscles while building up the hip flexors. It can also be used to help the student cultivate self-awareness as they work on their stability skills.

STEPS

1. Being in Staff Pose (p.91) with your legs extended in front of you and your hands on the floor, palms down, at your hips.
2. Tilt back slightly as you slowly raise both legs off the floor until they are at a 45 degree angle. Straighten your legs, point your toes, and swivel your upper torso to the left.
3. Place your left hand two feet or so behind your hip, palm down, as a support, and place your right hand between your thighs, palm down.
4. Cross your right foot over the left as you flex the left upward. Hold for three to five breaths before changing sides.

VARIATION

Prayer Hands: It is said that by performing Revolved Boat Pose with Prayer Hands, you will gain a sense of peace and unity. Balance on your tailbone and two sit bones, and bring your two hands to your chest, palms pressed together.

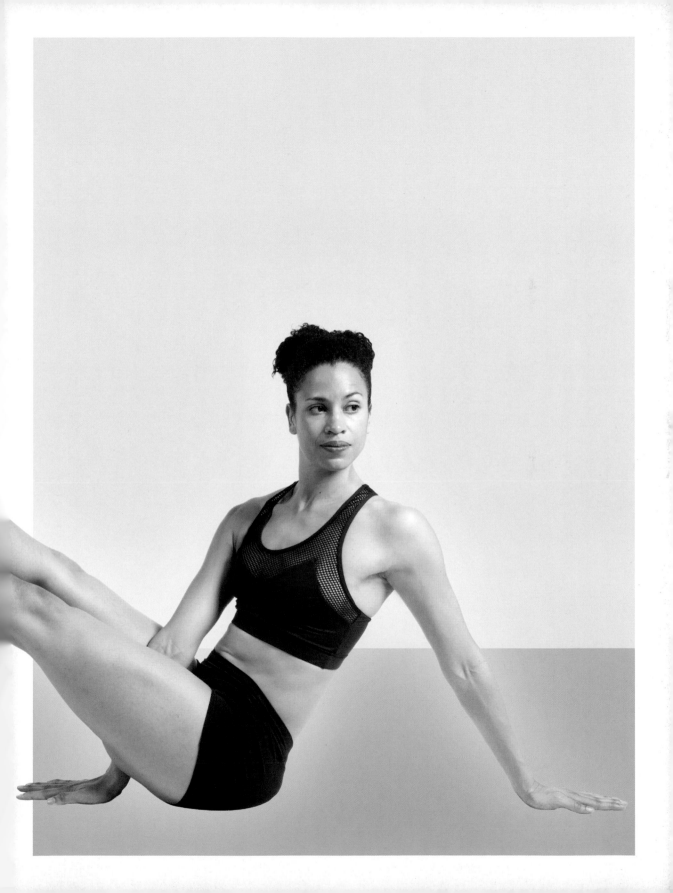

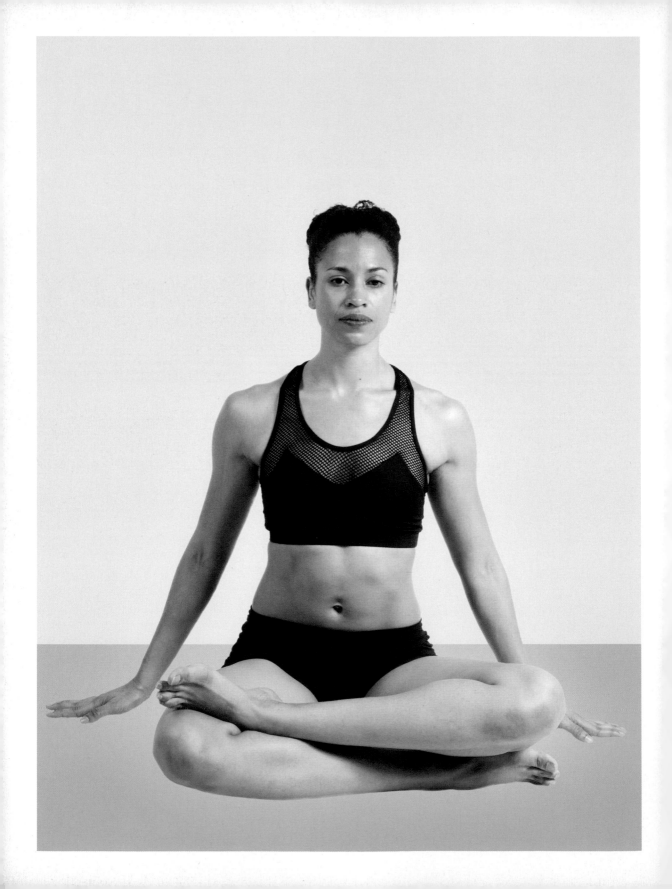

BEGINNER
INTERMEDIATE
ADVANCED

Half Lotus Pose

FIND YOUR FORM

Be sure to extend upward from the spine; keep breathing evenly throughout the pose.

BE CAREFUL OF...

Do not perform this pose if you have serious issues with your knees or hips.

This intermediate asana provides an excellent prep for the more demanding Full Lotus Pose. Also known as ARDHA PADMASANA, Half Lotus opens the hips and stretches the pelvis, legs, and ankles. Like any of the Lotus Poses, it should only be attempted near the end of a session, when you are thoroughly warmed up.

STEPS

1. Begin by sitting in Staff Pose (p.91) with legs extended and arms outspread beside you, hands palms down.
2. Bend your left knee, letting it fall open to the side until your thigh is on the mat.
3. Reach forward to grasp your left shin, and, as you rotate your hip outward, place your left foot upon your right thigh, the heel as close to your groin as possible.
4. Gentle ease your right foot beneath your left thigh. Then draw your knees together as you press your groin to the mat while keeping your sit bones stationary.
5. Place your hands on your knees, and hold the pose for three to six breaths before switching legs.

VARIATIONS

Firelog Pose: In this alternative Lotus prep, you sit with crossed legs, but keep the bottom leg on the floor and stack the upper leg across it so that your shins are parallel.

Elevated Half Lotus: Grasp a weighted Swiss ball in both hands and keep it elevated in front of you during the pose.

BEGINNER

INTERMEDIATE

ADVANCED

Full Lotus Pose

FIND YOUR FORM

Be sure to keep both soles facing up. Try to maintain the straightness in your back and upper body as you focus on extending your torso and easing stress from your mind.

BE CAREFUL OF...

Do not over extend your outer ankles or strain your knees. Do not allow your upper body to tilt to one side. Avoid this pose if you have hip, knee, or ankle issues.

PADMASANA may be the best known of all yoga poses, almost a cliché. Often associated with the practice of meditation, Lotus Pose opens the hips, stretches the lower body, and promotes balance and inner harmony. Although it appears simple, Full Lotus can be difficult to achieve and should be worked up to gradually.

STEPS

1. Begin in Easy Pose (p.90) with your legs crossed right over left, soles facing up. Grab your left shin and place your left foot so that it is resting on your right thigh. Position your right foot on your left thigh and draw the heel in toward your left hip. Work your ankles as far as you can up each thigh.
2. Flex your feet as you focus on keeping your knees and ankles in alignment. Rotate your hips externally and feel your inner knees roll away from each other.
3. Press your two sit bones to the floor to increase stability. With a neutral pelvis, draw your tailbone down toward the mat and your navel in toward your spine.
4. Elongate your torso and broaden your chest and colloarbones. Place your open hands on your knees, palms up for receiving energy or palms down to ground yourself.
5. Close your eyes as you hold the pose for three to five breaths before switching legs..

VARIATIONS

Prop Aid: If at first you have trouble sitting up straight, place a folded blanket under your hips to raise them above your knees.
Wisdom Pose: Create the classic gyana mudra—"wisdom" mudra—with your resting hands by connecting your forefingers and thumbs, palms facing your heart.

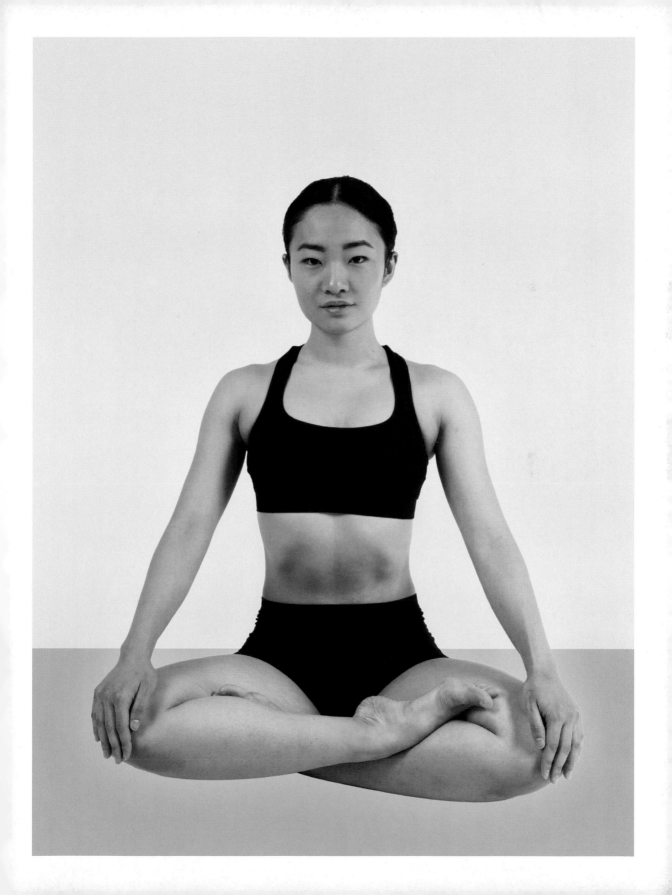

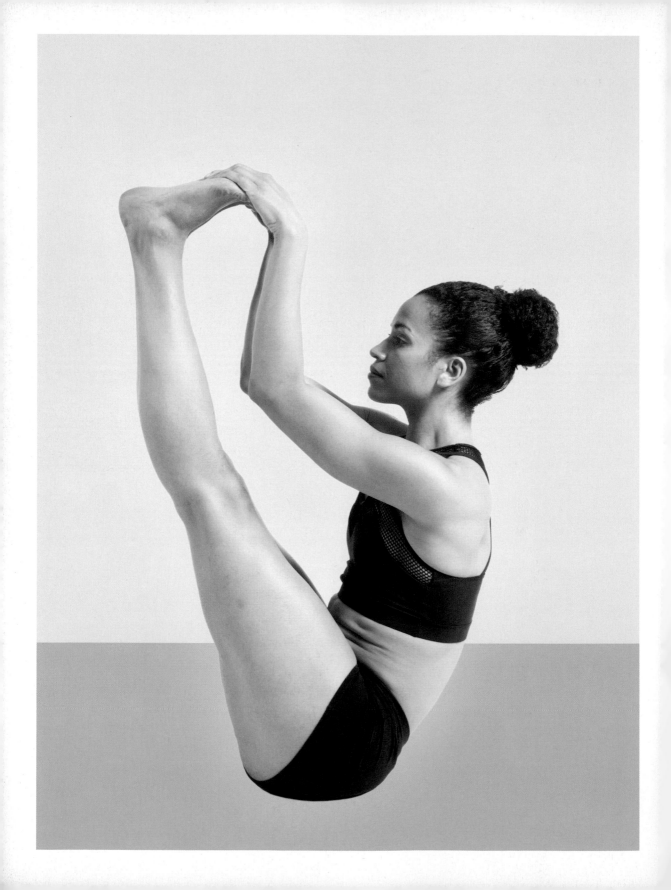

BEGINNER
INTERMEDIATE
ADVANCED

Big Toe Pose

FIND YOUR FORM

Be sure to keep your head and neck in neutral position, with your gaze forward, toward your raised shins.

BE CAREFUL OF...

Try not to rock back and forth when holding the pose. Avoid this pose if you have lower-back or ankle issues.

This advanced pose, called PADANGUSTHASANA in Sanskrit, can provide a stretch to the entire back of your body, including those often-tight hamstrings. As a balance pose it also builds up your stability and focus, works your core, and opens your arms, shoulders, and hips.

STEPS

1. Begin in Staff Pose (p.91) and draw both knees up toward your chest.
2. Tilt back slightly, and raise both legs until your shins are parallel to the floor.
3. Reach your hands out between your legs, and grasp your big toes firmly.
4. Once you are able to maintain balance, while sitting on your tailbone and two sit bones, slowly straighten both legs. Activate your abdominal muscles to increase stability. Press your toes with your fingers to flex your feet toward you.
5. Hold the pose for three to five breaths; repeat if desired.

VARIATION

Prop Aid: If at first you have difficulty grasping or straightening your legs, place a yoga strap across the soles of your feet and hold it taut.

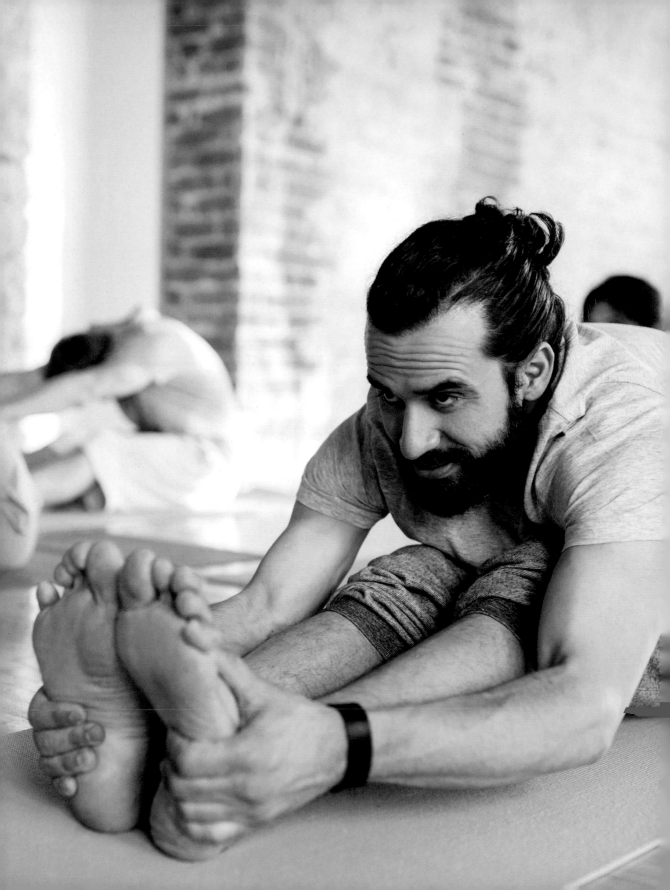

CHAPTER FOUR

Seated Forward Bends

Seated Forward Bends offer a deep stretch to the entire back of the body—the neck, shoulders, spine, buttocks, hamstrings, calves, and heels. These poses are also known to have a calming effect similar to that experienced during Standing Forward Bends. They can be effective for dealing with stress, mild depression, and headaches.

BEGINNER

INTERMEDIATE

ADVANCED

Child's Pose

FIND YOUR FORM

Release any tension you may feel in your body, especially in your facial or jaw muscles.

BE CAREFUL OF...

Try not to bring your knees too far apart. Avoid this pose if you have knee problems.

This relaxing, restorative beginner pose—with its passive stretching of the anterior muscles—can be assumed at any time during your session if you need to rest or regroup. Known as BALASANA in Sanskrit, it not only relieves back pain, it can also decrease levels of stress and anxiety.

STEPS

1. Begin by kneeling on your hands and knees in tabletop position with your arms shoulder-width apart.
2. Point your toes at each other, and move your knees to about hip-width apart.
3. Extend your torso toward the front as you shift your hips back toward your heels, and lower your stomach onto your thighs.
4. Lower your head, and round your shoulders until your forehead is resting comfortably on the floor.
5. Position your arms alongside your legs, palms facing up. Hold the pose for five to ten breaths...or as long as you require to feel renewed.

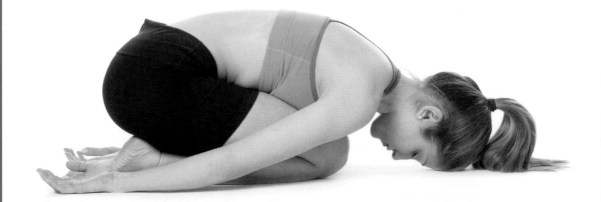

VARIATIONS

Extended Child's Pose: From Child's Pose, bring both arms forward, and stretch them out in front of you, palms pressed to the mat.

Prop Aid: Place a folded towel under your forehead if the head-down pose is uncomfortable.

BEGINNER
INTERMEDIATE
ADVANCED

Extended Puppy Pose

FIND YOUR FORM

Press down with your spread hands and lower legs and toes to keep yourself grounded. Keep your neck relaxed.

BE CAREFUL OF...

Do not let your lower back sink or your ribcage jut forward. Avoid this pose if you have knee or lower-back pain.

Downward Facing Dog, also known as ADHO MUKHA SVANASANA, is a restorative beginner pose known for relieving tight hamstrings, but it may need some working up to. Extended Puppy Pose, UTTANA SHISHOSANA, is an easier variation that can help new students avoid injury while they stretch their shoulders, lower torso, and legs.

STEPS

1. Begin by kneeling on all fours in tabletop position—hands positioned beneath your shoulders, knees below your hips, the tops of your feet on the mat.
2. Slide or walk your hands out in front of you until your arms are straight, shoulder-width apart, palms flat on the floor, fingers forward. To activate your arms, keep your forearms off the floor and your elbows lifted.
3. Exhale, and move your buttocks halfway back toward your heels as you lower your forehead to the floor.
4. Engage your abdominal muscles to support your lower back as you raise your hips and buttocks toward the ceiling.
5. Hold for five to ten breaths before returning to tabletop position.

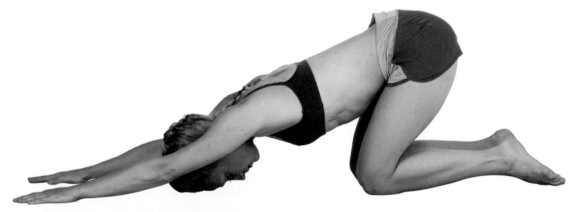

VARIATION

Prop Aid: To protect your lower back, activate leg and hips muscles by placing a rolled-up blanket between your legs.

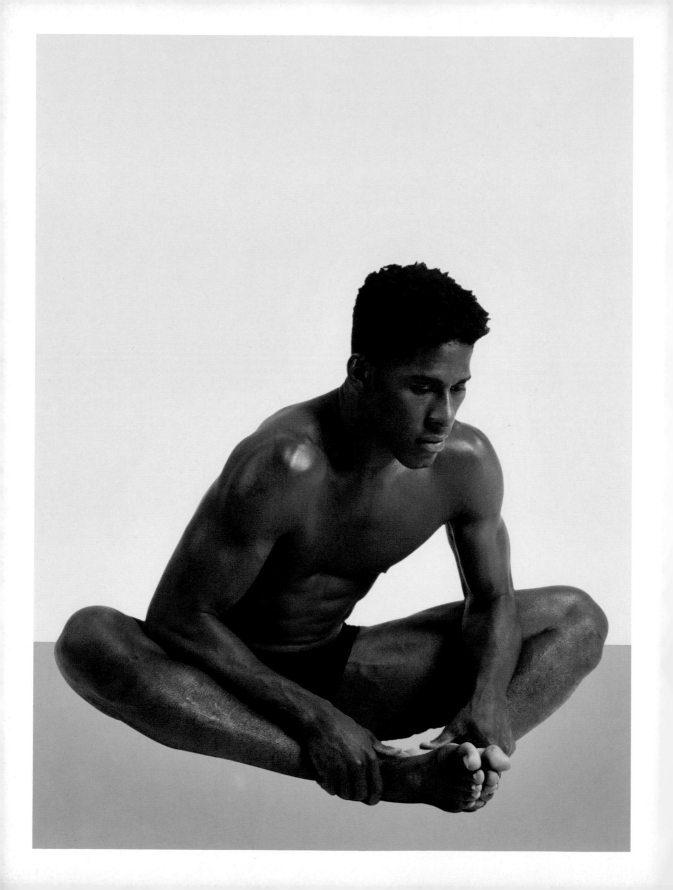

BEGINNER

INTERMEDIATE

ADVANCED

Bound Angle with Forward Bend

FIND YOUR FORM

Press your sit bones to the floor so that you don't rock on them or slouch as you bend.

BE CAREFUL OF...

Do not hold your breath during any portion of the pose. Avoid this pose if you have a groin or knee injury.

The Bound Angle Poses stretch the inner thighs, groin, and knees as well as opening the hips and increasing flexibility. They are known to relieve depression and ease menstrual cramping. By adding a forward bend to this asana, you can increase its benefits twofold.

STEPS

1. Begin by sitting upright on the mat with your knees bent and out to the sides and the soles of your feet pressed together.
2. Rest your elbows or forearms on your inner thighs and grasp the tops of your ankles with your hands. Draw both heels in as close to your groin as is comfortable.
3. On an exhale, tuck your navel in toward your spine, and lean your upper torso forward over your hands; continue forward until you feel a stretch in your groin.
4. Hold this pose for four to eight breaths.

VARIATIONS

Prop Aid: If you have trouble leaning over your feet, place a folded towel or cushion under your buttocks to elevate your hips.

Chin on Floor: Once this pose has you limbered up, try extending the forward bend until your chin is resting on the floor.

Arms Extended: From Step 3, release your ankles and place your extended arms on the floor in front of you, palms down.

BEGINNER
INTERMEDIATE
ADVANCED

Seated Forward Bend Prep

FIND YOUR FORM

Make sure you concentrate on elongating your torso as you bend.

BE CAREFUL OF...

Keep breathing normally during this pose. Avoid performing it if you have lower-back issues.

This beginner pose will help you to achieve a really deep bend when you finally attempt the intermediate-level Seated Forward Bend. The pose can increase the flexibility and mobility of your back, hamstrings, and calves, and allow you to really extend your torso.

STEPS

1. Begin by sitting straight up on the floor with your legs extended and parallel. Relax your feet, and flex them slightly.
2. Rest your forearms or hands on your knees.
3. Hinge forward from your hips until your abdomen is over your thighs. Keep your back as straight as possible.
4. Hold this pose for four to eight breaths before easing up into sitting position. Repeat if desired.

VARIATION

Prop Aid: If your calves or hamstrings feel stiff, slip a yoga band over the balls of your feet and tug it toward your hips to help increase your bend.

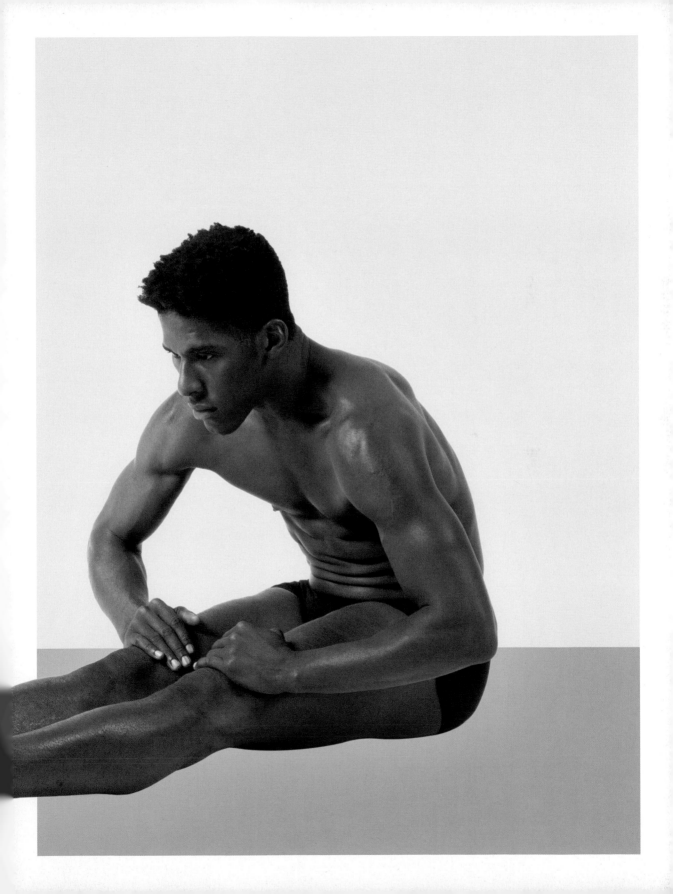

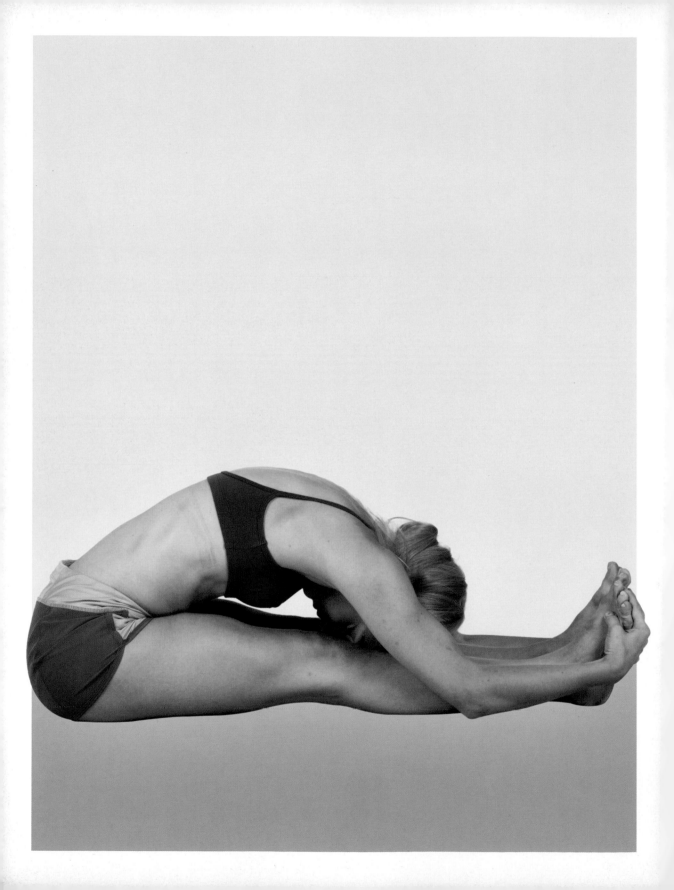

BEGINNER
INTERMEDIATE
ADVANCED

Seated Forward Bend

FIND YOUR FORM

Make sure your big toes are not flexing toward you more than the other toes. Your feet should be at right angles to your body, as though your were standing.

BE CAREFUL OF...

Never force yourself into a deep bend; keep practicing until you are able to stretch naturally. Avoid this pose if you have lower-back or hamstring issues.

Also known as PASCHIMOTTANASANA in Sanskrit, the intermediate Seated Forward Bend requires a great deal of lower body and leg flexibility. But it's worth the work—this asana stretches the spine, shoulders, and hamstrings and also stimulates the liver, kidneys, ovaries, and uterus.

STEPS

1. Begin by sitting in Staff Pose (p.91) with your feet slightly flexed. Raise your arms above you, parallel to each other, as you sit up tall and elongate your torso.
2. On an exhale, lean forward from the hips, and bring your hands down to your ankles.
3. Clasp the sole of each foot with the corresponding hand, keeping your elbows or forearms on the mat.
4. Fold your abdomen down over your thighs as your head comes to rest gently on your shins.
5. Hold for four to eight breaths; as you breathe, lengthen your exhalations until they are longer than your inhalations.

VARIATION

Western Intense Stretch: To release the lower back, from Forward Bend Pose raise both arms, and grasp your toes as you sit up slightly with your head between your arms. Flex your toes forward, and straighten your arms, as you again lower your head to your shins.

BEGINNER
INTERMEDIATE
ADVANCED

Head-to-Knee Forward Bend Prep

This beginner pose make a good precursor to the intermediate-level Head-to-Knee Forward Bend. It will free up tight hamstrings and calves, placing more difficult bends within your reach; it is also known to ease digestive problems.

FIND YOUR FORM

If your back feels stiff or tight, try doing the pose with a sofa or armchair behind you, and keep your lower back in contact with the prop.

BE CAREFUL OF...

Avoid this pose if you suffer from lower-back problems.

STEPS

1. Begin by sitting in Staff Pose (p.91) with your legs parallel and outstretched in front of you, toes pointing forward.
2. As you bend your left knee, let it fall to the outside, and place the sole of your left foot on your inner right thigh slightly above your knee.
3. Lean forward from the hips over your right thigh; with your elbows wide, place your meshed hands or forearms on your right knee.
4. Hold for four to eight breaths before switching to the other side.

VARIATION

Intense Stretch: Increase the benefits of this stretch, especially to your rhomboids, by lowering your head as you bend forward.

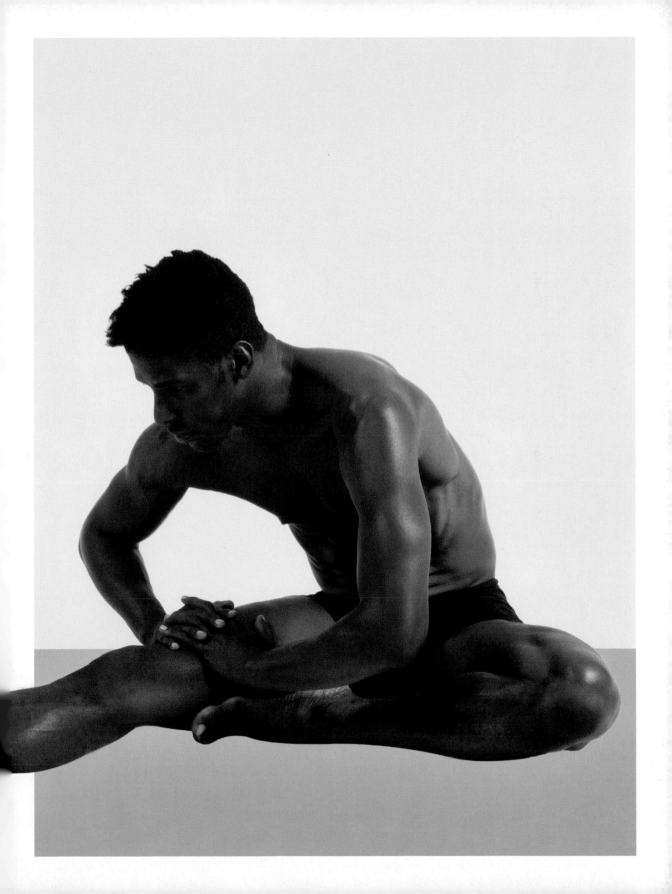

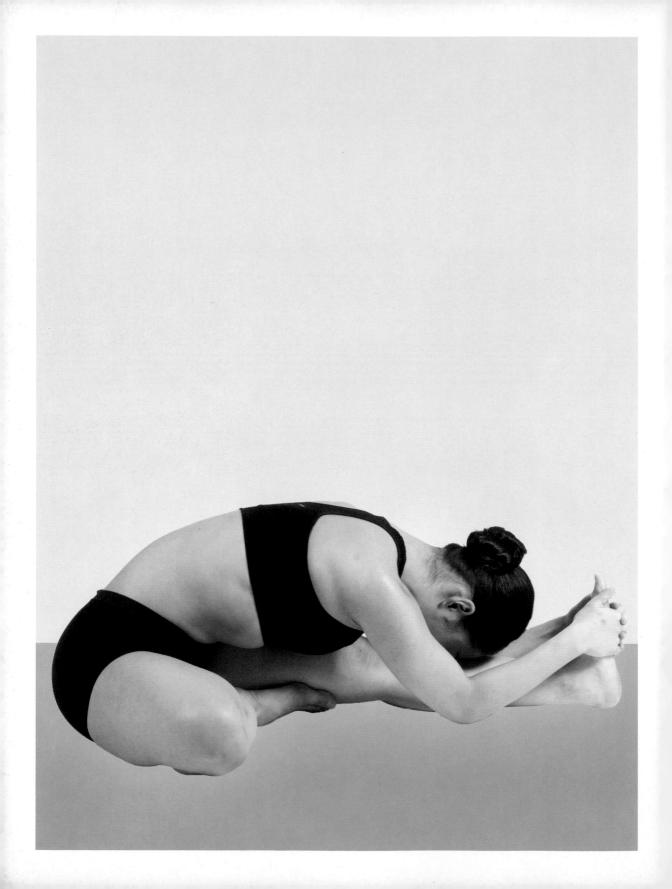

Head-to-Knee Forward Bend

FIND YOUR FORM

Fold down gradually onto your leg with your abdomen, then your chest, then your forehead.

BE CAREFUL OF...

Do not let your back round as you bend; don't allow your tucked foot to push under your thigh. Avoid this pose if you have knee or lower-back issues or are suffering from diarrhea.

This intermediate forward bend, JANU SIRSASANA, offers a host of benefits—it not only stretches the spine and lower body, it can also help to combat fatique, reduce anxiety, soothe headaches, aid digestion, and even ease painful menstruation.

STEPS

1. Begin sitting in Staff Position (p.91) with your legs outstretched and feet flexed.
2. Keeping your knee on the floor, bend your right leg and tuck the sole of your right foot against your left thigh until your right shin is perpendicular to your left leg.
3. Elevate your chest and spine with an inhale, then pivot until your torso aligns with your left leg.
4. On an exhale, draw your abdomen in, and bend forward over your left thigh.
5. Reach forward with both hands to grasp your left foot— or place both hands flat on the floor, elbows bent, on either side of your foot.
6. Lower your forehead to your left shin; hold for three to six breaths before repeating on the other side.

VARIATION

Prop Aid: You can assist your forward bend by sitting on a folded blanket or low cushion.

BEGINNER
INTERMEDIATE
ADVANCED

Revolved Head-to-Knee Pose

FIND YOUR FORM

Be aware of all the tension created by this pose: the elbows in opposition; the torso and spine bent and twisted; the supporting knee bent; the foot and thigh in active contact; the extended foot flexed.

BE CAREFUL OF...

Do not allow your shoulders to round or hunch as you bend and twist. Avoid this pose if you have lower-back or knee issues.

Also called PARIVRTTA JANU SIRSASANA in Sanskrit, this versatile intermediate pose creates a deep side stretch, works the shoulders, spine, and hamstrings, and stimulates digestion. Approach it only when you are thoroughly warmed up and at your most limber.

STEPS

1. Being sitting in Staff Pose (p91) with legs outstretched, toes flexed.
2. Move your right leg slightly to the right. Bend your left leg, and tuck your left sole against your upper right thigh. Externally rotate your right thigh.
3. Hinge to the right, and place your right forearm on the inside of your right shin; reach with your right hand to grasp the sole of your foot,
4. Reach up with your left arm, externally rotate it from the shoulder, then reach down to grasp the top of your right foot. Your elbows should be opened away from each other.
5. Tuck your right shoulder against your right thigh, and lean back, twisting to angle your right ribs toward the ceiling. With your head centered between your arms gaze forward, and hold for three to five breaths.

VARIATION

Extended Arm: For a less intense pose, bend slightly to the side over your extended leg, place your right hand on your right shin, raise your left arm beside your left ear, and gaze up at your raised palm.

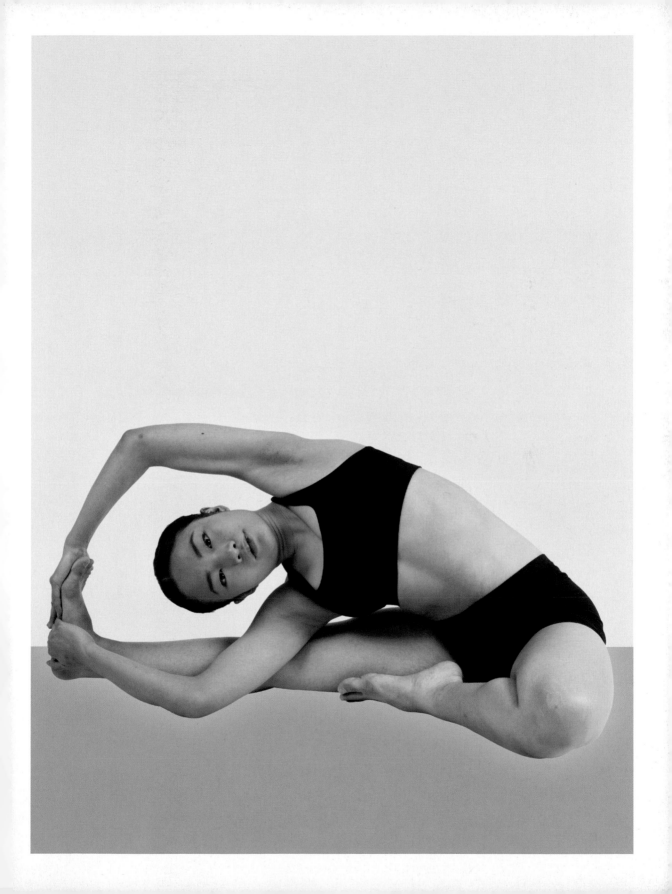

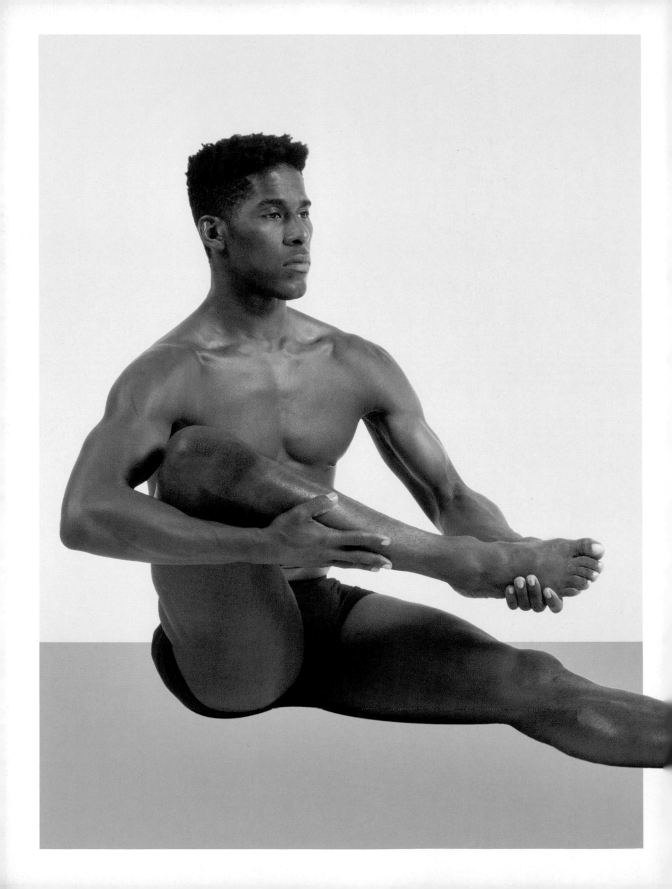

BEGINNER

BEGINNER
INTERMEDIATE
ADVANCED

Seated Cradle Leg

FIND YOUR FORM

Keep your chest open and your gluteal muscles active as your raise your shin.

BE CAREFUL OF...

Do not attempt this pose if you have groin or hip injuries.

This intermediate pose is a great way to tone and stretch your gluteal muscles as well as your hips and hamstrings. Known as HINDOLASANA in Sanskrit, it is also used to ease the lower-back tension or stiffness suffered by those who sit all day at a desk or computer.

STEPS

1. Being sitting in Staff Pose (p.91), sitting upright with legs extended and feet flexed.
2. Bend your right knee and slide your heel up close to your groin.
3. With your right hand grasp your calf and raise your leg. Clasp your right heel or the outer edge of your foot with your left hand.
4. Draw your shin toward your chest, cradling it like an infant. Make sure to keep the foot at least 12 inches from your chest to avoid knee injury.
5. Hold for three to five breaths before repeating on the other side.

VARIATION

Foot Tuck: If it is more comfortable at first, you can tuck your left sole under your right thigh before lifting the right leg.

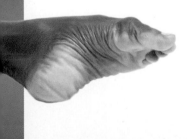

Side-Leaning Half Straddle Pose

FIND YOUR FORM

Lean from your hips; imagine that your raised hand is reaching for your extended knee.

BE CAREFUL OF...

Don't allow you buttocks to leave the floor; keep your sit bones grounded. Avoid this pose if you have a groin injury or issues with your lower back.

This intermediate pose, also known as SAMAKONASANA, offers a deep stretch to the oblique muscles of the side as well as to the core and legs. It can help decompress your spine after a long day at the office, open your groin, and improve the flexibility of your hips and leg joints.

STEPS

1. Sitting upright in Staff Pose (p.91), bend your left knee and draw your left sole against your right thigh. Extend your left leg out as far to the side as is comfortable with toes pointed.
2. Place your hands, palms down, on the floor behind your hips. This is basic Straddle Pose.
3. Bend you right elbow and bring your forearm to rest on your inner right thigh.
4. Lift your left arm up toward the ceiling, palm facing inward. Let your gaze follow your hand. Bend to the right without crunching forward—until you feel a distinct stretch in your sides.
5. Keep your gaze forward and neck neutral as you hold for three to six breaths before switching sides.

VARIATION

Elbow Down: For an even greater side stretch, place the elbow of your lowered arm on the floor in front of your inner thigh.

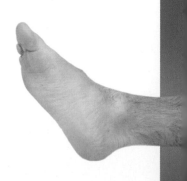

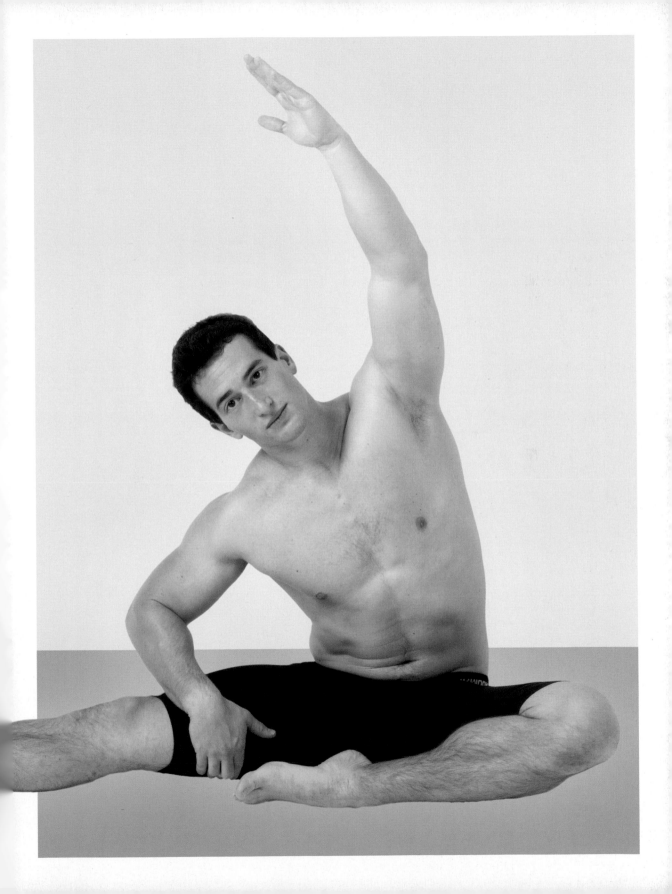

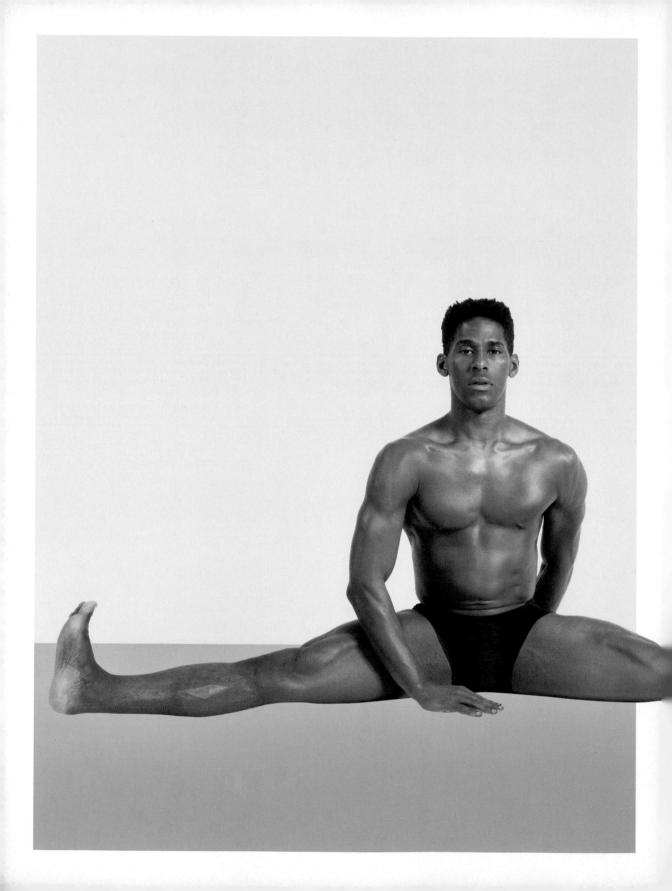

Seated Straddle Split Pose

FIND YOUR FORM

Sit up tall and resist the urge to lean back or round your shoulders.

BE CAREFUL OF...

Never bounce your legs to force them wider apart; with practice, your split will soon widen. Avoid this pose if you have groin or hips issues.

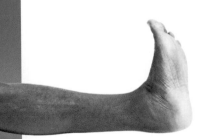

This demanding intermediate pose, called KONASANA, requires that you have already learned to bend from the hips and maintain your balance on the tripod of your tailbone and two sits bones. It increases hip and hamstring flexibility, tones the glutes and inner thighs, and opens the groin.

STEPS

1. From Staff Pose (p.91) spread your legs out as wide as is comfortable. Rotate your thighs slightly outward so that your knees are facing up; flex your feet, heels pushing out.
2. Place both hands behind your buttocks to help push them forward.
3. Then place one hand behind you and the other directly in front of you to support your torso as you square your hip bones.
4. Sit up tall and focus on sending energy down through your legs to your toes. Hold for three to five breaths before switching hands.

VARIATIONS

Floor Lift: To increase the difficulty, press your palms to the floor, and slightly raise your body from the mat. Slowly bring your pelvis forward. Hold for three to five breaths. Repeat three times.

Chest to Thigh: From Seated Straddle Split, place your hands on either side of your extended knee, twist you torso, and lower your chest over your thigh.

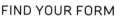
Chest-to-Floor Straddle Split

FIND YOUR FORM

Be sure to keep your knees facing up to the ceiling. Elongate your back as you lower your torso to the floor; do not let it round.

BE CAREFUL OF...

Do not bend forward from your waist; instead, hinge at your hips. Avoid this pose if you have groin or lower-back issues.

VARIATION

Prop Aid: If you have trouble bending forward from your hips or spreading your legs wide, sit on a folded blanket to elevate your hips.

Also called the Wide-Angle Seated Bend, or UPAVISTHA KONASANA in Sanskrit, this intermediate/advanced pose stretches the groin and hamstrings while strengthening the spine. Remember not to force your legs or body into any pose that is painful; a discernible stretch is what you are seeking.

STEPS

1. Begin by sitting in Staff Pose (p.91). Turn your legs outward a bit so that your knees face the ceiling, and flex your feet.
2. Spread your legs as wide apart as is comfortable. Place your hands, palms down, behind your buttocks to push them forward and open your groin even farther.
3. On an inhale, elevate your torso as you place your hands on the floor in front of you. Tighten your leg muscles, and press the backs of your thighs and your sit bones into the floor.
4. Carefully slide your hands out in front of you as you hinge your torso forward from your hips. Keep your gaze forward as you reach as far as you can without rounding your back.
5. Hold for three to six breaths before easing upright.

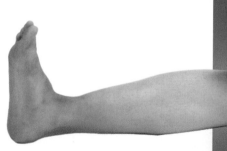

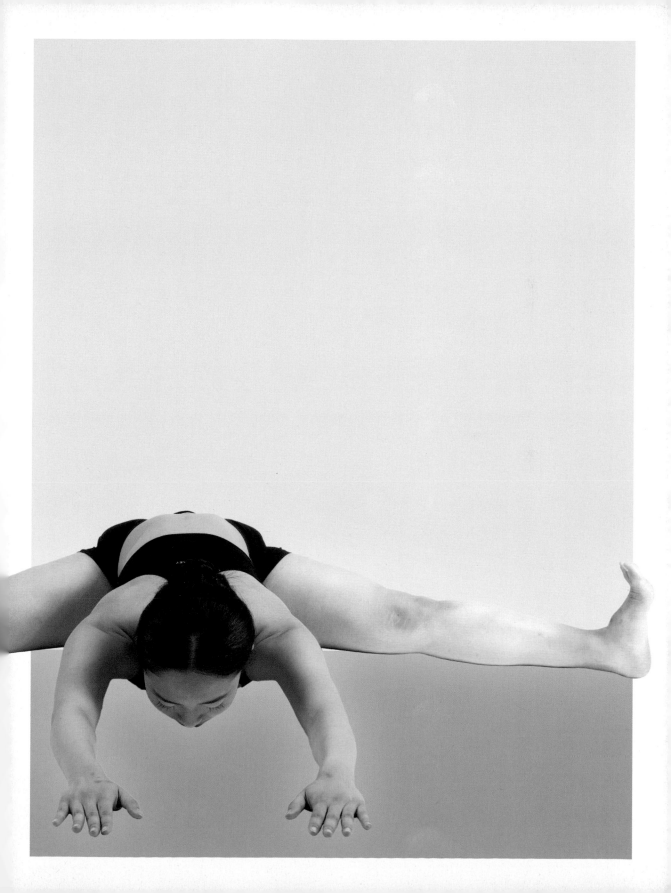

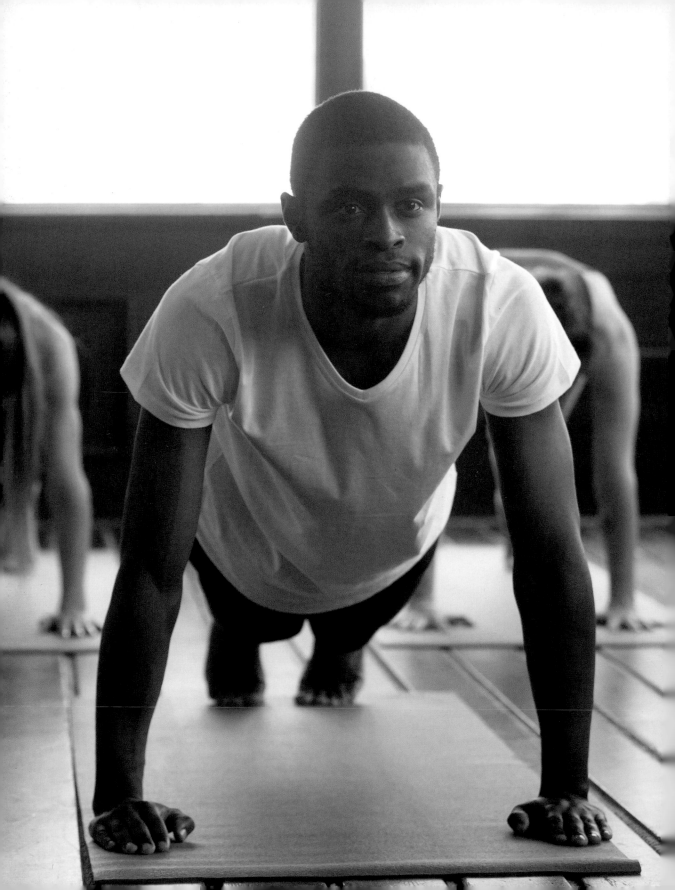

CHAPTER FIVE

Arm Supports

Arm Supports utilize the weight of your body to increase their strength-building effects on the arms, wrists, hands, and shoulders, while providing an effective stretch to the sides, buttocks, and legs. They offer deep toning for the abdomen, which is called upon to provide stability during these poses. If you spend hours working at a desk or computer, they can help to unknot the tension found in your neck, shoulders, and collarbone.

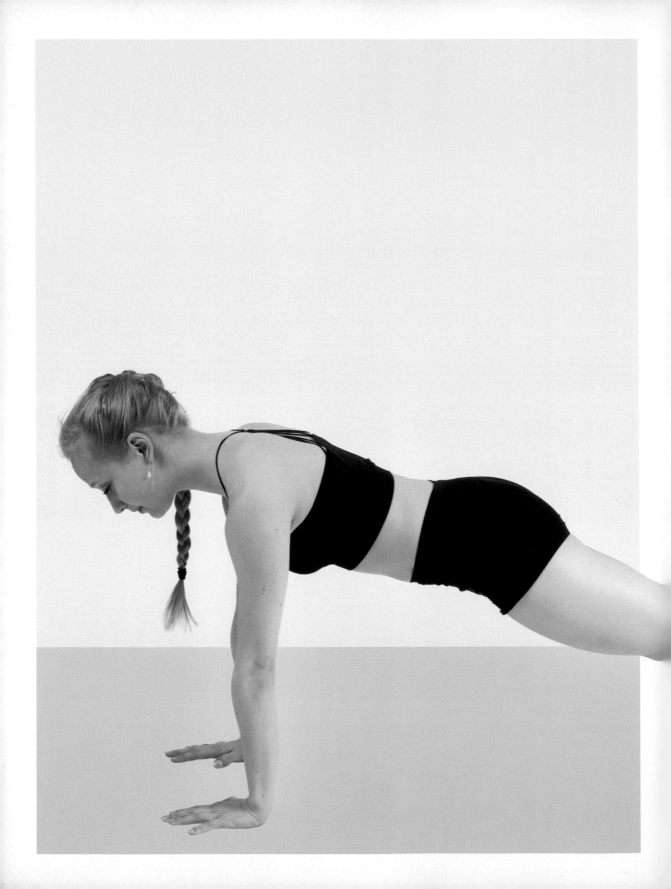

BEGINNER
INTERMEDIATE
ADVANCED

Plank

FIND YOUR FORM

Be sure to broaden across your collarbones as you soften your upper back between your shoulder blades. Your wrists should be squared to the front of your mat.

BE CAREFUL OF...

Do not lift your fingers from the floor—press them down for grounding. Avoid this pose if you suffer from wrist, shoulder, or elbow injuries.

The Plank Poses elevate the upper body by using the arms while keeping the lower limbs more earthbound. The basic beginner Plank tones the stomach, arms, and wrists, and offers a good prep pose for more intense arm-supported asanas. Plank Pose is often included in yoga sequences.

STEPS

1. Begin in Downward-Facing Dog (p.191) with your arms straight and shoulder-width apart.
2. Shift your torso forward so that your shoulders are now positioned above your wrists. With arms parallel, rotate your elbows externally until the inner part of your elbows faces forward.
3. Raise up onto the balls of your feet; spread your toes to ground them as your heels push back.
4. Your body should now form an almost straight line from your shoulders, through your spine, to your heels. Rotate your thighs inward, and keep them taut; lengthen your lower spine toward your heels.
5. With your head in neutral position, hold for four to eight breaths.

VARIATION

One-Legged Plank: While in hold, raise your buttocks slightly and lift one leg to hip height—or higher—with the toes pointed and your sole facing up.

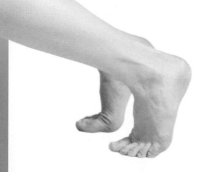

BEGINNER

INTERMEDIATE

ADVANCED

Chaturanga Pose

FIND YOUR FORM

Tightened glutes and abs will help stabilize your core. Keep your hips at the same level as your shoulders, not lower.

BE CAREFUL OF...

Do not let your elbows bend to the extent that your chest sinks or your shoulders round. Avoid this pose if you have shoulder, elbow, or wrists problems.

VARIATION

Take a Knee: If maintaining this pose is still too hard at first, kneel out of Plank Pose, then bend your elbows and lower your torso to just one or two inches off the floor.

Also known as the Four-Limbed Staff Pose, this beginner asana is usually referred to by its Sanskrit name. This popular plank, which focuses on strengthening the arms, wrists, abdomen, and legs, as well as honing balance, is often incorporated into flows and sequences.

STEPS

1. Begin in Plank Pose (p.140) with your arms straight, your body extended, and palms and the balls of your feet grounded on the floor.
2. On an exhale, bend your elbows and lower your torso until your upper arms are parallel to the floor with your elbows tucked close to your side.
3. Ground yourself through your palms as you tuck in your abdomen and draw your tailbone down to keep your lower back from drooping. Move your shoulder blades together to keep your shoulder tips away from the floor.
4. Keep your neck long, and gaze just beyond the front edge of the mat as you hold for three to six breaths.

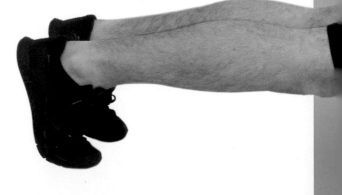

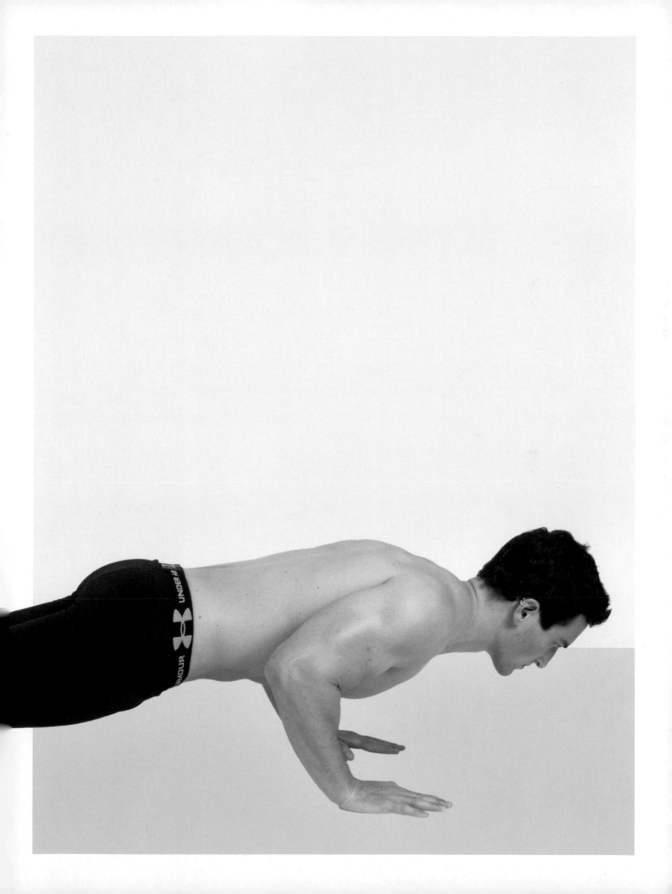

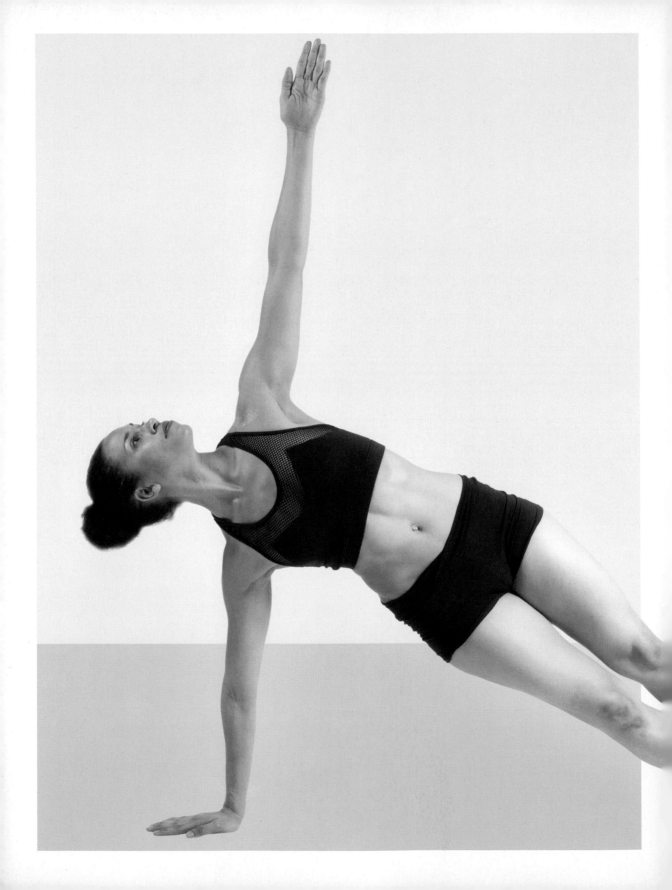

BEGINNER

INTERMEDIATE

ADVANCED

Side Plank

FIND YOUR FORM

It helps to elongate you arms and legs as much as you can.

BE CAREFUL OF...

Do not bring your hips up too high; don't allow them or your shoulders to sink or sway. Avoid this pose if you have shoulder, elbow, or wrists issues.

This rather challenging beginner pose, also known as VASISTHASANA, strengthens the upper body, abdominals, and legs, while it stretches the obliques and shoulders. It also provides a great way to work on your balancing skills. The real test is maintaining straight alignment in your legs and torso

STEPS

1. Begin in Plank Pose (p.140) with arms straight, body extended, and weight grounded on your palms and the balls of your feet.
2. Shift your weight to the outside of your right foot and to your right hand and arm.
3. Stack your left foot on top of your right foot, and press them together, with both feet flexed.
4. On an exhale, raise your left arm straight up toward the ceiling, fingers outstretched.
5. Turn your face up and shift your gaze to your raised fingers. Hold for three to five breaths before switching to the other side.

VARIATION

One-Legged Side Plank: While in hold, rotate your hip outward, and raise your top leg until it is parallel to the floor. If you are really limber, raise it up toward your elevated hand and grasp your toes. For less difficulty, bring your foot to your knee.

INTERMEDIATE

ADVANCED

Dolphin Plank

Also known as MAKARA ADHO MUKHA SCANASANA, this valuable beginner plank is an isometric pose that builds lean muscle while strengthening your abdominals and the backs of your legs and stretching your shoulders, upper arms, and obliques.

FIND YOUR FORM

As with the other plank poses, tightened abs and glutes help maintain a straight line through your torso and legs. Keep your shoulder blades and collarbones wide (in preparation for balance poses like Crane or Crow).

BE CAREFUL OF...

Don't poke your buttocks into the air, which reduces the load on your muscles. Avoid this pose if you suffer from shoulder injuries or abdominal strain.

STEPS

1. Begin on all fours in tabletop position, with your toes curled forward.
2. Bend your elbows, and place your forearms on the floor shoulder-width apart, palms down.
3. Raise your knees off the ground and extend your legs behind you until they are in line with your torso.
4. Ground yourself with your forearms and the balls of your feet pressed to the mat.
5. Keep your neck relaxed in neutral position as you gaze toward the front of the mat; hold for three to five breaths.

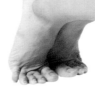

VARIATIONS

One-Legged Dolphin: To increase intensity, while in hold raise one foot off the ground for several breaths, then switch to the other foot.

Arm Reach: While in hold, reach one arm straight out to the side, palm down for several breaths.

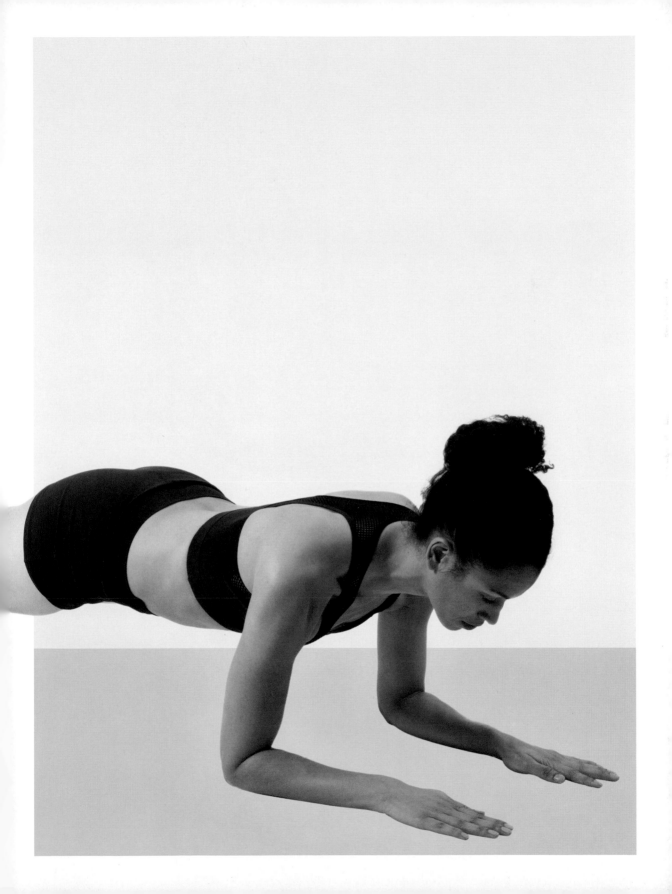

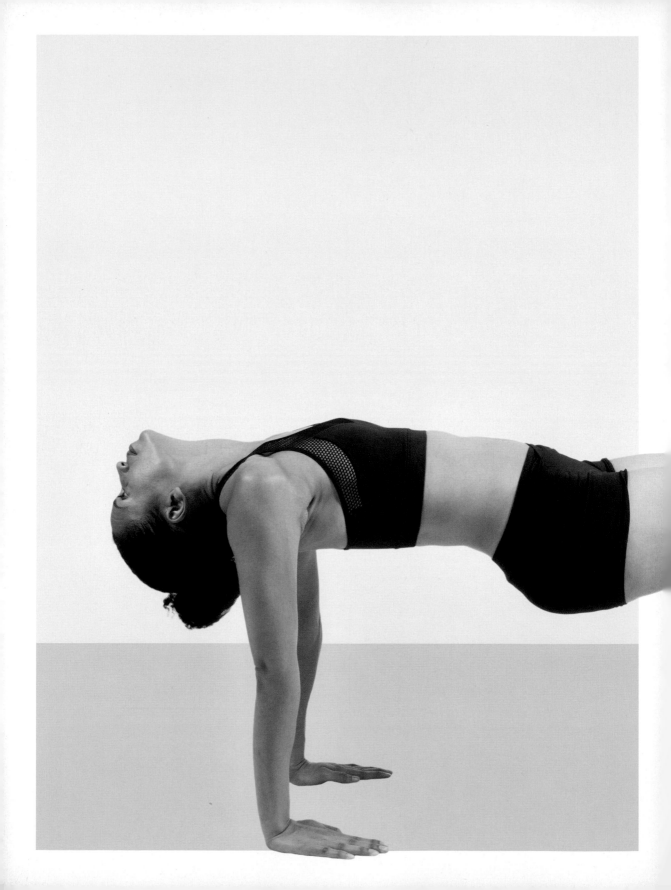

BEGINNER
INTERMEDIATE
ADVANCED

Reverse Tabletop Pose

FIND YOUR FORM

During the final pose, your entire torso should be as parallel to the floor as possible..

BE CAREFUL OF...

Do not lean your head too far back; a neck position should never be painful. Avoid this pose if you have lower-back issues or a wrist injury.

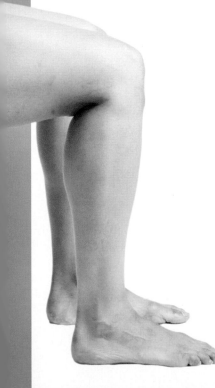

This position is also referred to as Crab Pose, Half Upward Plank Pose, or ARDHA PURVOTTANASANA. It is especially useful as a counterpose to performing forward bends. It stretches your quads and hamstrings while strengthening your upper back and glutes. As a chest opener, it energizes your body and corrects your posture.

STEPS

1. Begin in Staff Pose (p.91) with your legs in front of you. Press your palms to the mat just behind your hips, fingers pointing forward. Bend your knees, and press your soles to the mat.
2. Grounding yourself with your palms and soles, tighten your buttocks and thighs. and raise your torso up so that your hips are even with your knees. Your shins should now be perpendicular to the floor and your wrists should be directly below your shoulders
3. Expand your chest as you draw your should blades together.
4. Keep your neck in neutral position, or tip your head back slowly until you can gaze beyond the back of your mat.
5. Hold the pose for three to five breaths, easing the tension in your buttocks and letting your legs do the lifting.

VARIATION

One-Legged Crab: On an inhale, raise one leg to hip height as you press down with the grounded foot.

BEGINNER
INTERMEDIATE
ADVANCED

Upward-Facing Plank

FIND YOUR FORM

Use your hamstrings and shoulders, not your back, to expand your hips and chest. Widen your legs if your hamstrings complain.

BE CAREFUL OF...

Do not let your head loll back. Don't let your ribcage jut or your buttocks droop. Avoid this pose if you have issues with your wrists, elbows, shoulders, or neck.

VARIATION

One-Legged Reverse Plank: While in hold, raise one leg to hip height while pressing down with the grounded foot.

This intermediate pose, called PURVOTTANASANA in Sanskrit, takes the Reverse Tabletop into full plank mode. It is effective for building up arm, leg, and back muscles, and for stretching the chest, abdominals, ankles and feet. As a balance pose, it also improves your stability.

STEPS

1. Start by sitting upright in Staff Pose (p.91). Place your hands eight to ten inches behind your hips, fingers facing forward.
2. Bend your knees, and press your soles to the mat with your heels no less than 12 inches from your buttocks. Turn your toes slightly inward.
3. On an exhale, press down with your palms and soles as your raise your hips to knee level; your back and thighs should be parallel to the floor, your wrists directly below your shoulders.
4. Extend your legs along the mat one at a time while keeping your hips and spine elevated. Lift your chest, and draw your shoulder blades together until there is a slight hollow in your back.
5. Drop your neck back until you can gaze up at the ceiling; hold for three to five breaths.

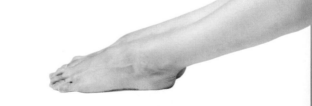

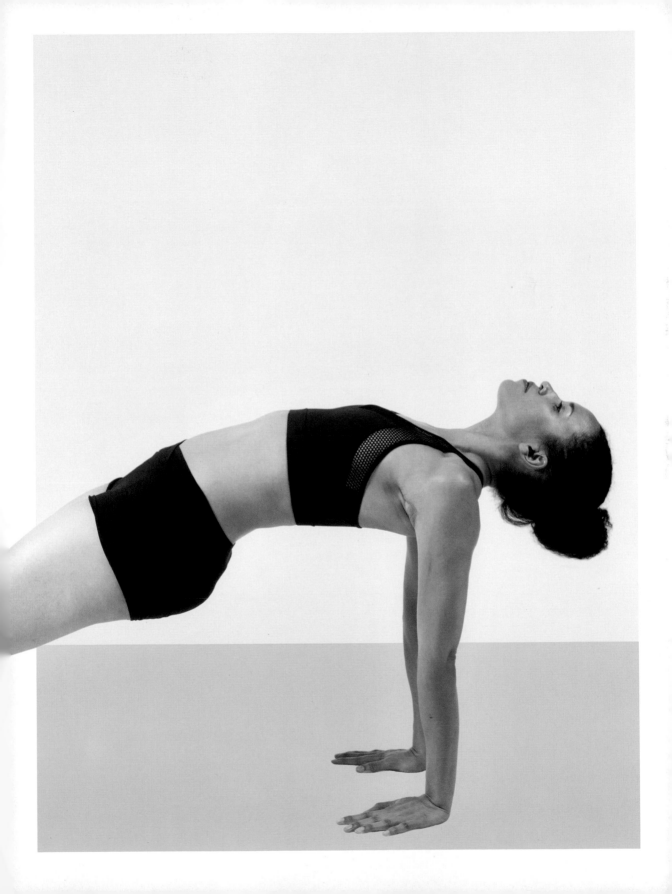

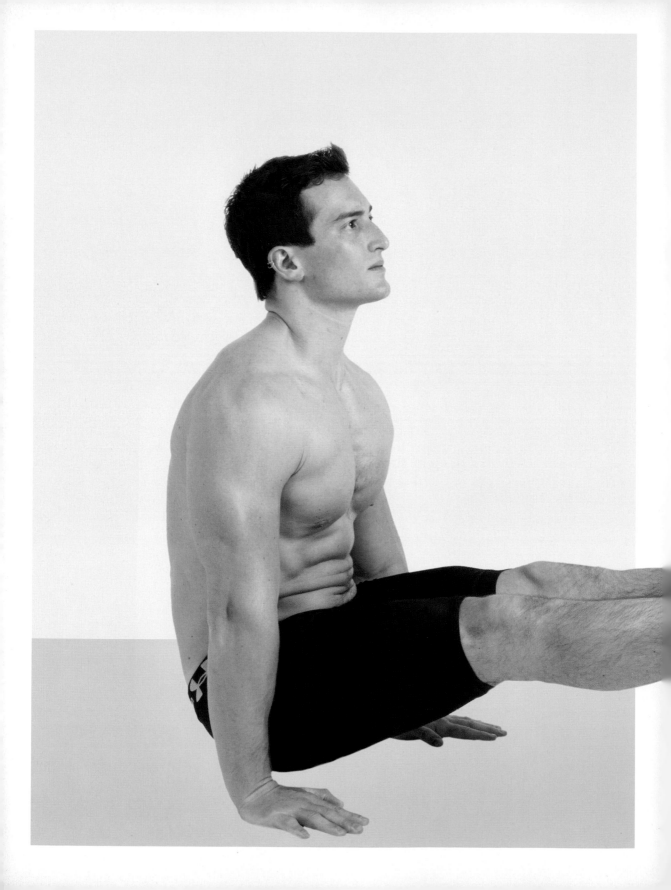

Celibate Pose

FIND YOUR FORM

Try to keep your legs together and straight by engaging your abdominal, thigh, and buttocks muscles.

BE CAREFUL OF...

Do not allow your shoulders to hunch or round while in pose. Avoid this pose if you suffer from wrist or shoulder issues.

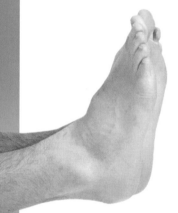

This intermediate pose, also called BRAHMACHARYASANA, offers a great way to strengthen your abdomen, pelvis, shoulders, and quads. Its Sanskrit name refers to exerting control over one's senses, especially sexual desire, which is where the English name derives from.

STEPS

1. Begin sitting upright in Staff Pose (p.91) with your legs outstretched.
2. Place your palms beside your hips, elbows straight, palms flat on the mat.
3. Activate your legs, abdomen, and chest, keeping them taut.
4. On an inhale, press down with both hands—they may move up or back as you find your center of gravity—and raise your torso and legs off the ground, bearing the weight with your arms and shoulders. The strength required to perform this will occur over time even if it seems difficult at first.
5. Hold the pose for as long as is comfortable, then lower yourself down on an exhale. Repeat several times.

VARIATION

Prop Aid: If you initially cannot lift your body clear, sit on the mat, and practice raising your legs in the proper position.

BEGINNER
INTERMEDIATE
ADVANCED

Crow Pose

FIND YOUR FORM

To maintain balance, it helps to gaze at one spot on the floor below you.

BE CAREFUL OF...

Never hop into a balance pose. Go slowly and carefully, raising one foot off the floor at a time. Avoid this pose if you have wrist issues.

There is some confusion between Crow Pose and Crane Pose; both are challenging, two-handed balance poses, but Crow (KAKASANA) is performed on bent arms, while Crane (BAKASANA) is performed on nearly straight arms. They work admirably to strengthen the arms, abdomen, and wrists.

STEPS

1. Begin in Garland Pose (p.26), squatting with your feet more than hip-width apart.
2. Lean forward, and place your hands on the mat, fingers facing slightly inward. Bend your elbows deeply and then, rising on the balls of your feet, press your knees against the outside of your upper arms.
3. "Climb" your arms with your knees as you bring your thighs closer to your chest. Seek your center of gravity as you tip forward on both hands, and raise one foot at a time.
4. Once you feel your entire weight transfer to your wrists, round your back.
5. Hold the pose for as long as is comfortable.

VARIATION

Crane Pose: While holding a strong Crow Pose, tuck your thighs against your torso, shift your knees to the backs of your forearms, pressing them hard, and try to straighten your elbows.

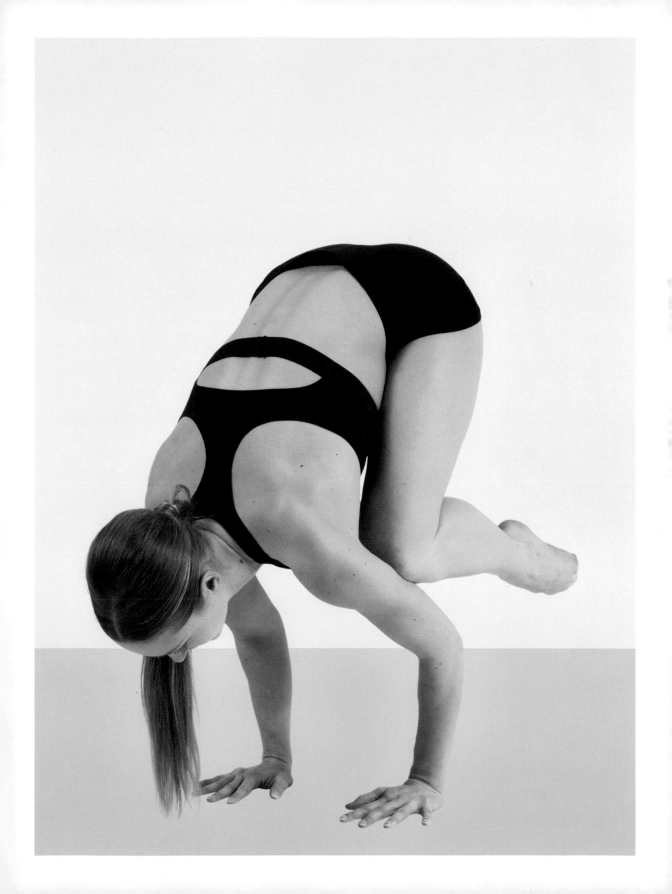

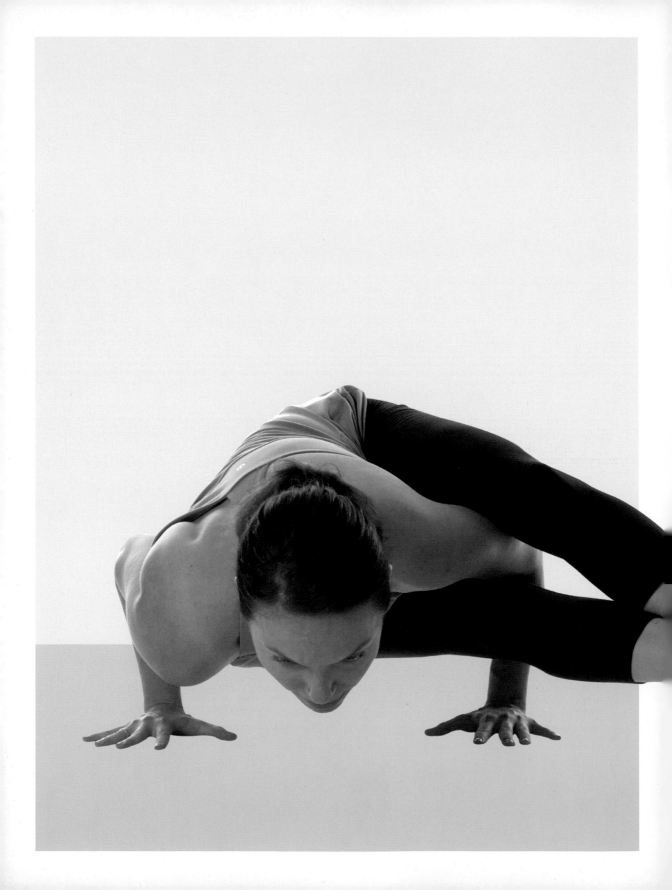

BEGINNER

INTERMEDIATE

ADVANCED

Eight-Angle Pose

FIND YOUR FORM

Remember to twist your legs together more from the spine than the hips.

BE CAREFUL OF...

Do not allow your upper hip to dip back, which will make the lower hip drop. Avoid this pose if you have shoulder, elbow, or wrist issues.

This advanced asymmetrical balance pose, known as ASTAVAKRASANA, works several different muscle groups—those in your shoulders, arms, and torso, as well as those found in the back of your thighs and calves. It is also a good way to hone your balancing skills.

STEPS

1. Start sitting upright in Staff Pose (p.91) with your legs extended and you arms down at your sides, palms on the floor.
2. Lift your left leg until the thigh is perpendicular to the floor. Slip your left arm under your bent knee so that your left calf is just below your left shoulder.
3. Press both hands to the floor beside your hips and bend your elbows as you lean forward, raising your torso up from the mat.
4. Straighten your right leg in front of you, and exhale as you level your torso. Swing your right leg to the left and, bending both knees, twine your ankles around each other.
5. Press your legs together, and angle them to the left as you shift your torso to the right.
6. Hold for as long as is comfortable before repeating on the other side.

VARIATION

Leg Lift: Until you feel capable of the final ankle twist, you can keep your lower leg straight in front of you as you raise yourself off the mat.

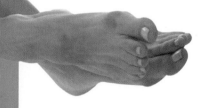

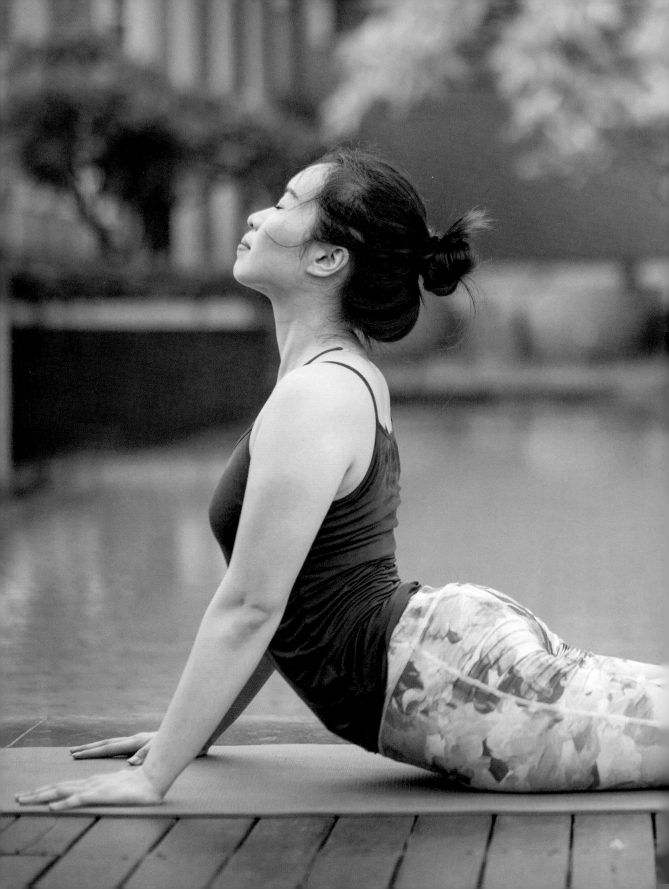

CHAPTER SIX

Backbends

Yoga backbends consist of any pose where the spine is curved backward. This position engages the abdominal muscles, the obliques, and the leg muscles, which all help to steady the student while the pose is being held. Backbends offer a number of therapeutic benefits, such as opening the chest and shoulders, but they are especially useful for addressing back issues.

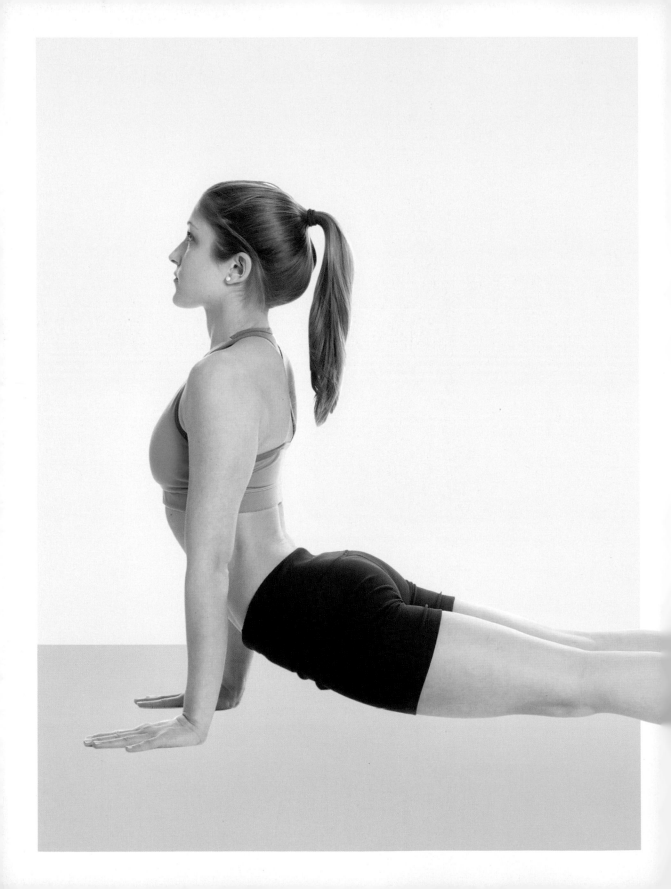

BEGINNER

INTERMEDIATE

ADVANCED

Upward-Facing Dog

FIND YOUR FORM

It helps to imagine there is a line of energy running diagonally through you, from the lower tips of your shoulder blades to your collar bones in order to open up your chest.

BE CAREFUL OF...

Avoid this pose if you have a headache, are pregnant, or have injuries to the wrist, hand, neck, shoulders, or low back.

This popular pose strengthens the wrists, arms, and back, while it opens the chest and heart and counteracts "office slump." Considered an extroverted pose, it balances the human tendency to curl in on ourselves when depressed or stressed. Upward-Facing Dog is often performed in tandem with Downward-Facing Dog; both are found in most Sun Salutations and Vinyasas.

STEPS

1. Lie facedown on the mat; bend your elbows, keeping them tight to your sides, and place your palms on the mat below your shoulders. Spread your legs to hip-width apart with your toes facing back.
2. On an inhale, press down with your palms and the tops of your feet; lift your torso and hips off the floor.
3. Tighten your thighs as you tuck your tailbone down toward your groin.
4. Raise yourself up through your chest by straightening your arms and arching your back. As you press your shoulders down and back, extend your neck to gaze ahead and slightly upward.
5. Hold for three to six breaths before lowering yourself down.

VARIATION

Toes Curled: For extra attention to the upper body and core, perform this pose with your legs elevated off the floor and your toes curled forward.

BEGINNER

INTERMEDIATE

ADVANCED

Cobra Pose

FIND YOUR FORM

Take your time extending up into cobra. As you improve, try moving your planted hands slightly behind your shoulders. Note that in Cobra Pose, unlike Upward-Facing Dog, only the upper part of the torso is raised and the elbows remain bent.

BE CAREFUL OF...

Take care that you don't strain your neck in this pose; remember that your back should be doing all the work. Avoid this pose with lower-back issues or if you are pregnant.

VARIATION

Extended Cobra: Plant your hands in front of you and straighten your elbows almost completely as you arch into a deep backbend, your head back, your gaze on the ceiling.

Cobra Pose, or BHUJANGASANA, is one of the most effective yoga poses for stretching the spine, shoulders, and abdomen. Considered a moderate backbend, it opens up the chest and strengthens the back. Child's Pose makes a good counterpose after performing Cobra.

STEPS

1. Lie facedown with your legs extended behind you, hip-width apart and the tops of your feet on the floor.
2. Bring your hands to the sides of your ribs positioned beneath your elbows.
3. Spread your fingers wide, keeping your elbows bent and close to your body. Let your weight fall to your wrists and hands as you lift your upper torso off the floor until your chest and upper abdomen are no longer touching the ground.
4. Lift your crown toward the ceiling as you raise up, and hold this pose for five to eight breaths.

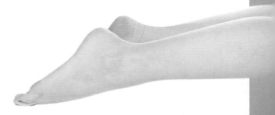

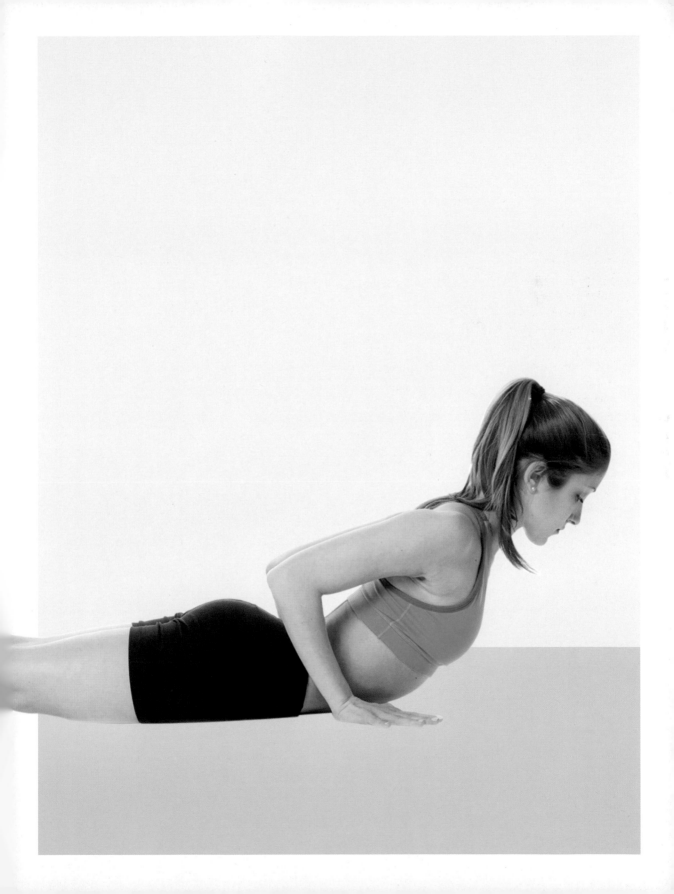

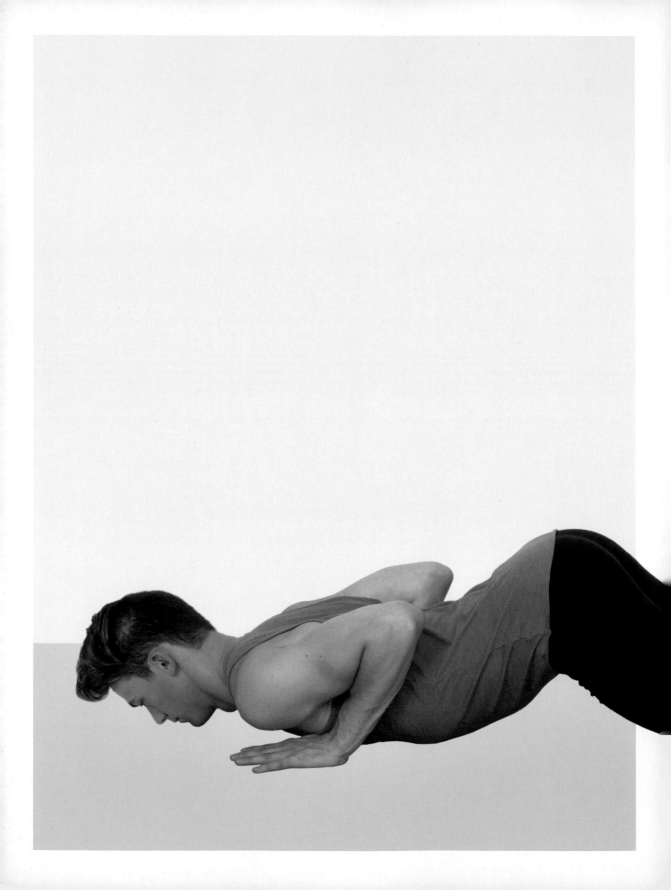

Knees-Chest-Chin Pose

FIND YOUR FORM

Make sure to maintain a hollow in your spine and a dip between your shoulder blades.

BE CAREFUL OF...

Avoid this pose if you have shoulder or abdominal pain.

Also known as ASHTANGPRANAMA, this strength-building transitional pose makes a great preparation for full-body weight-bearing poses such as planks. It is also an element of the Sun Salutations and is often used as a warm-up. The pose focuses on the core, shoulders, chest, arms, and back; it can stimulate the abdominal organs and relieve stress.

STEPS

1. Begin by kneeling on all fours, your arms positioned below your shoulders, knees a foot or so behind your hips. Curl your toes forward.
2. Bend your elbows and keep them close to your ribcage
3. Round your spine into a concave arch as you lower your chest and chin to the ground. Your shoulders and chest should align with your hands. Your elbows and buttocks should be reaching up.
4. Hold for three to six breaths.

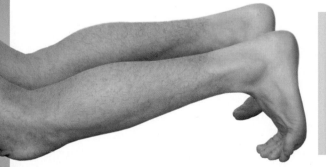

VARIATIONS

Prop Aid: You can place a folded towel beneath your chin for comfort.
Low Cobra: From final pose, push with your toes to move forward onto your stomach as you arch your back and rise into a low Cobra Pose.

BEGINNER
INTERMEDIATE
ADVANCED

Bridge Pose

FIND YOUR FORM

Keep your hamstrings taut to activate your legs; the bend should come from your shoulders and upper back, not your lower back.

BE CAREFUL OF...

Do not stick out your stomach or ribs or clench your buttocks. Avoid this pose if you have shoulder, neck, or back issues.

This beginner pose makes an excellent prep for full-lift backbends like Wheel Pose. Also known as SETU BANDHA SARVANGASANA, Bridge is a restorative pose that stretches the chest and spine, strengthens the buttocks and thighs, stimulates digestion and the thyroid gland, and relieves stress.

STEPS

1. Begin lying faceup on the floor, knees bent with your heels drawn up below your knees and your arms along your sides, palms down.
2. On an exhale, press down with your soles as you raise your buttocks off the floor.
3. Press down into your arms and palms as you raise your hips until the rest of your torso is off the floor; your spine should create a graceful concave arch from thighs to shoulders.
4. Extend your neck beyond your shoulders as you gaze upward. Hold for three to five breaths.

VARIATIONS

Prop Aid: Place a yoga block under your sacrum if you need the support at first.
One Legged Bridge: To increase the intensity, bend your elbows, and prop up your hips with your hands as you raise one leg up to the ceiling, toes pointed.

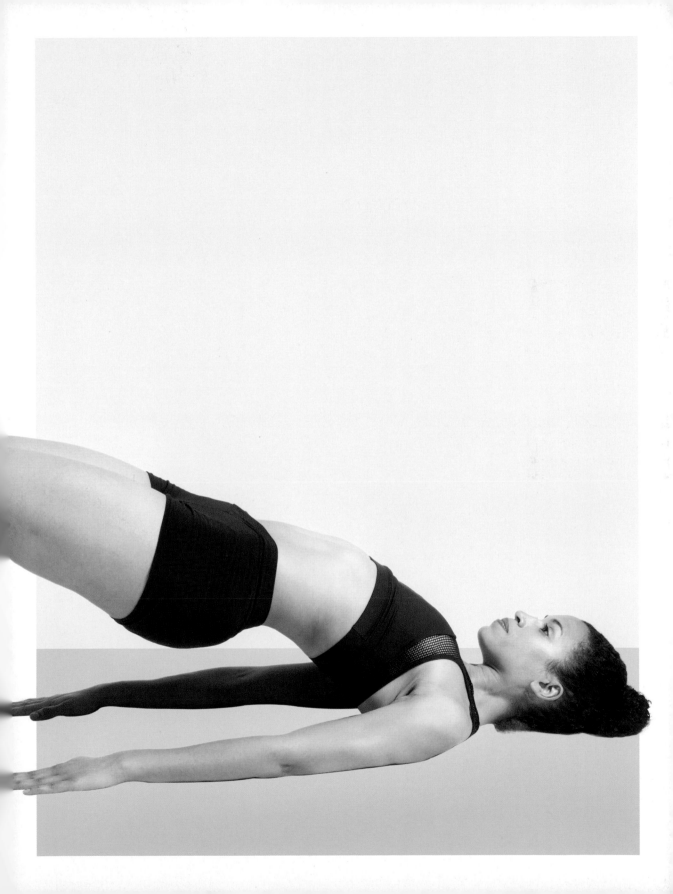

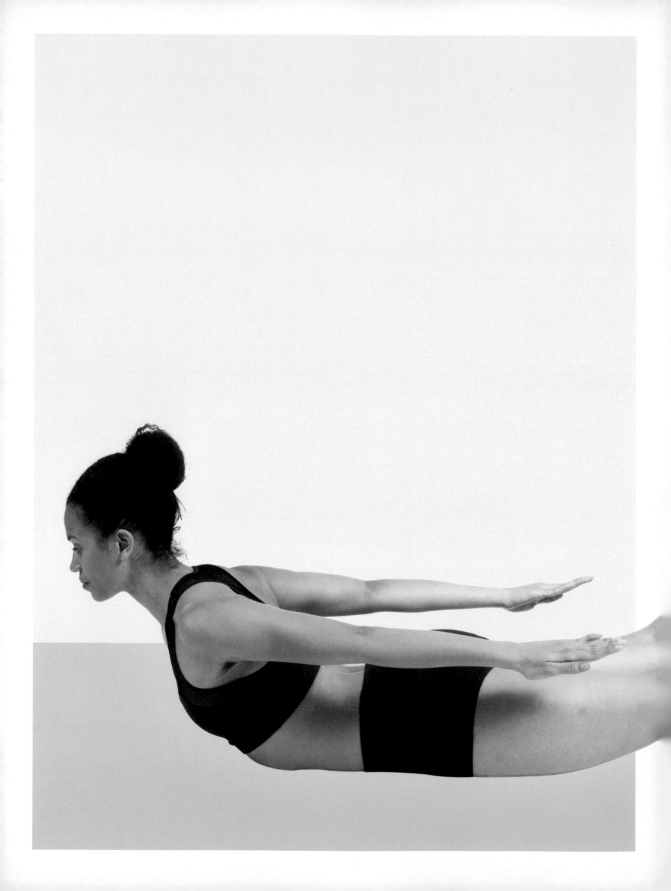

BEGINNER
BEGINNER

INTERMEDIATE

ADVANCED

Locust Pose

FIND YOUR FORM

By opening your chest, you can extend the bend throughout your back. Breath at a slow, steady rate.

BE CAREFUL OF...

Do not allow your knees to bend. Avoid this pose If you have back or uterine issues, blood pressure problems, or are pregnant.

Also referred to as Grasshopper Pose, or SALABHASANA or SHALABHASANA in Sanskrit, this beginner/intermediate pose targets the lower back, chest, and neck muscles, tones the abdominal muscles, stimulates the internal organs, and improves posture and menstrual function. Use it as a prep for deeper backbends such as King Pigeon and Lord of the Dance.

STEPS

1. Lie on your stomach with your chin on the mat, arms reaching back, palms down, and your feet hip-width apart. Turn your knees in slightly to face the floor

2. On an inhale, tighten your buttocks by pressing your pubic bone to the floor as you raise your head, arms, chest, and legs from the mat into a gentle arc. Keep your abdominals engaged to stabilize your center.

3. Extend your arms, palms flat, by reaching as far behind you as possible, keeping them parallel to the floor.

4. Keep you neck in neutral position; hold for three to five breaths.

VARIATION

Half Locust Knee Bent: From Locust Pose, bring your arms up and out as if preparing to dive, then bend the left leg and raise the knee from the floor while the right leg remains grounded. Hold for several breaths, then switch legs.

Half Frog Pose

Also known as ARDHA BHEKASANA, this intermediate backbend is a useful precursor before attempting the more demanding Bow Pose. It stretches much of the body—shoulders, neck, torso, abdomen, hips, thighs, and ankles—as well as strengthening the back.

FIND YOUR FORM

Make sure your hips and shoulders each remain level throughout the pose. Use your abdominal muscles for balance and support.

BE CAREFUL OF...

Do not sink into your supporting shoulder or twist your neck. Avoid this pose if you have lower-back or shoulder issues or have high or low blood pressure.

STEPS

1. Begin lying facedown on the mat with your forearms and the tops of your feet on the floor. Bend your elbows up and position your hands, palms down, on either side of your ribs. Keep your elbows tucked in close.
2. On an inhale, press down into your hands as you raise your upper torso from the floor. Keep your pubis pressed down to keep your core stabilized.
3. Bend your right knee, and draw your heel toward your right buttock. Shift your weight onto your left hand, and reach back with your right hand to grasp the inside of your right foot.
4. Rotate your wrist so that your fingers are facing forward as your press the top of the right foot, easing it closer to your buttock.
5. Increase the stretch by moving your right foot to the outside of your right hip with the sole facing the floor.
6. Bring your head upright, and gaze forward; hold for three to five breaths before switching sides.

VARIATION

Bent Elbow Half Frog: If at first you can't support your torso on your straightened arm, lower yourself down onto your forearm and elbow.

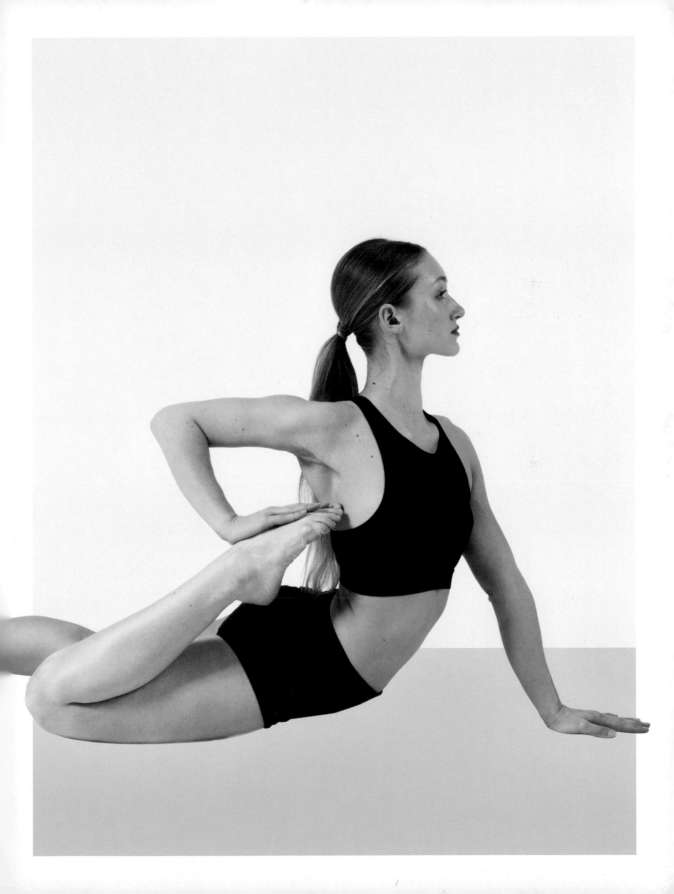

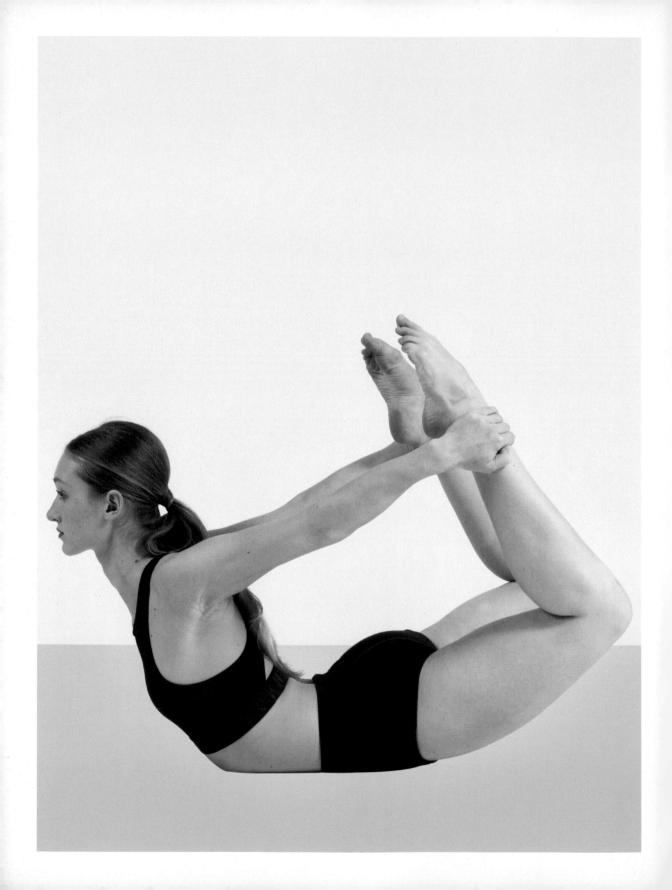

Bow Pose

This intermediate pose, called DHANURASANA in Sanskrit, strengthens and stretches almost the entire body, including the shoulders, arms, back, chest, abdomen, hips, groin, thighs, and ankles. It is also effective for improving circulation and aiding digestion.

FIND YOUR FORM

Draw your shoulder blades together to help open your chest. Make sure to raise your chest and thighs at the same time.

BE CAREFUL OF...

Do not externally rotate your thighs; you want the inner thighs rotating toward the ceiling. Avoid this pose if you have lower-back, shoulder, or knee issues or you are pregnant.

STEPS

1. Begin lying facedown with your forehead on the mat, legs hip-width apart, and your arms straight behind you at your sides.
2. Press your pelvis and lower abdomen into the floor to create a stable base for the pose. Bend your knees and bring your calves up over the backs of your thighs.
3. On an inhale, reach back with straight arms and grasp the outsides of your ankles.
4. On an exhale, raise your chest and thighs up from the mat, creating a concave arch in your spine. Draw your feet away from your shoulders to increase the lift in your chest.
5. Internally rotate both thighs, and tuck your tailbone down to ease any pressure on your lower back.
6. Balance on your lower abdomen as you equalize the extension between the lift of your chest and of your legs. Keep your gaze forward as you hold for three to five breaths.

VARIATION

Toe Flex: For additional stretch in your calves, flex your feet while in hold.

BEGINNER
INTERMEDIATE
ADVANCED

Upward-Facing Bow Pose

FIND YOUR FORM

While in hold, extend your tailbone down toward your knees, while raising your front hipbones toward your ribs.

BE CAREFUL OF...

Do not let your thighs rotate externally; this can compress your lower spine. Avoid this pose if you have elbow, knee, neck, back, or wrist issues or if you are pregnant.

Also called Upward-Facing Bow Pose or CHAKRASANA or URDHVA DHANURASANA in Sanskrit, this intermediate asana provides a deep, energizing backbend. It strengthens the whole body, opens the chest and ribs, and improves posture. It is also effective for easing asthma, combating osteoporosis, and relieving depression.

STEPS

1. Begin by lying on your back with you knees bent. Position your feet hip-width apart and, on an inhale, raise your arms up, palms forward. Bend your elbows and place your hands down next to your ears, fingers facing your feet.
2. Press into the mat with your palms and soles as you raise your hips to knee height and rest your crown on the floor.
3. Rise up into a true backbend while straightening your elbows as you rotate the inner part of the upper arm inward. Press down with all four corners of your feet as your weight shifts to your heels.
4. Rotate your inner thighs toward the mat and allow your head to hang down in a comfortable position between your arms. Hold for three to five breaths.
5. To release the pose, shift your body weight to your shoulders as you bend your arms and descend.

VARIATION

Supported Wheel: At first, you may want to try getting into position by placing a bolter under your back before arching up. Or even a bolster on three yoga blocks, which would raise you even higher.

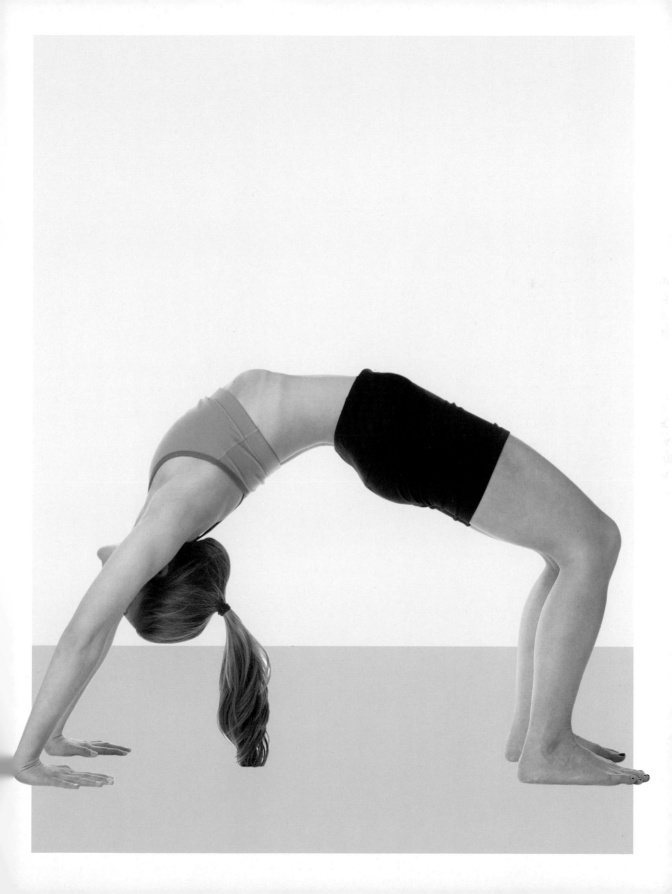

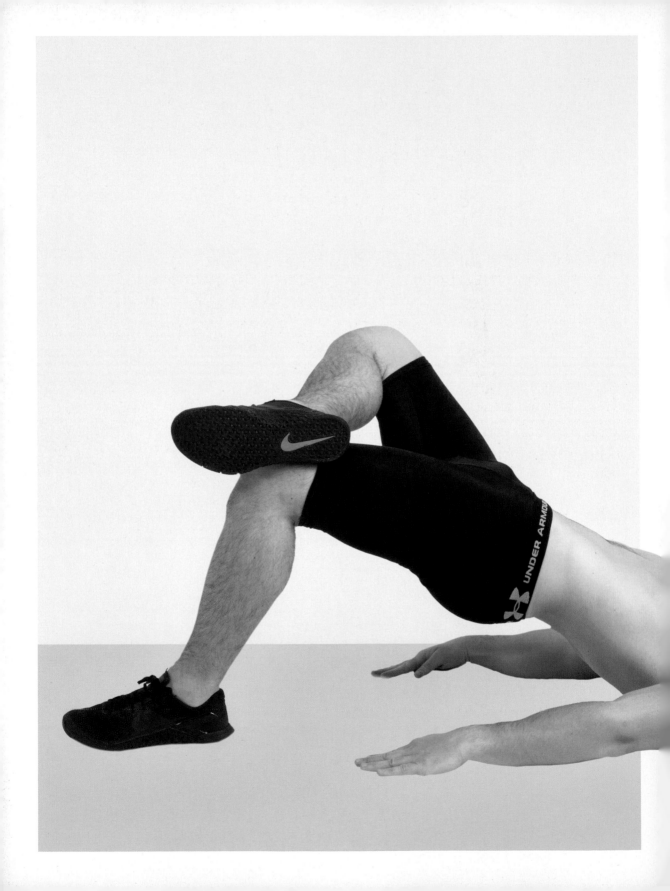

BEGINNER
INTERMEDIATE
ADVANCED

Bridge Pose, Eye of the Needle

FIND YOUR FORM

Anchor yourself with your arms, and tighten your buttocks and draw your navel toward your spine for stability. Keep your neck relaxed.

BE CAREFUL OF...

Don't allow your shoulders to creep up to your ears; press them down toward your back. Avoid this pose if you have shoulder, back, or neck issues.

This intermediate pose focuses on one of the gluteal muscles, the piriformis. Rotating your hip and turning your leg and foot outward while raising your torso, provides a deep muscle stretch, one that also stimulates digestion, relaxes tension, and tones the core.

STEPS

1. Start by lying faceup on the mat with your arms at your sides, knees bent, and soles flat on the floor.
2. Raise your right leg and slide your outer calf over your left knee.
3. Press your palms and toes down to the mat while you tighten your abdominals and buttocks. Lift your torso from the floor so that it forms a diagonal from your supporting knee to your shoulders.
4. With your gaze on the ceiling, hold for three to five breaths before lowering your torso with control. Repeat on the other side.

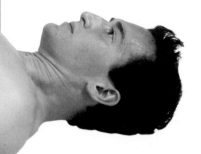

VARIATION

Ankle Stretch: While in hold, try flexing your raised foot forward and back to increase the stretch in your ankle and Achilles tendon.

Camel Pose

FIND YOUR FORM

While bending back, remember to keep your thighs perpendicular to the floor.

BE CAREFUL OF...

Try not to bend from your hips or drop your head too far back. Avoid this pose if you have knee, lower-back, or neck issues.

The intermediate position known as Camel Pose, or USTRASANA, opens the chest and shoulders and stretches the abdomen, thighs, and hip flexors. It is also a good way to improve your posture and relieve a stiff back or neck from hunching over a keyboard or too much texting on a cell phone.

STEPS

1. Begin by kneeling upright, with your arms relaxed and your knees hip-width apart.
2. Bend your elbows, and bring your hands to your hips. Draw your elbows together to open your chest, and internally rotate your thighs. Press down on your buttocks with your hands as you extend your torso up from your lower back.
3. Gently bend from your upper back, and reach behind you with straightened arms to touch your heels. Meanwhile, keep your chest expanded and your collarbones broad.
4. Let your head drop back slightly, keeping your gaze ahead. Hold for three to five breaths, then release the pose by raising your head and torso, and fold down into Child's Pose.

VARIATION

Arm Support: For a less-intense version of the pose, before bending back, place your hands behind your hips rather than reaching for your heels.

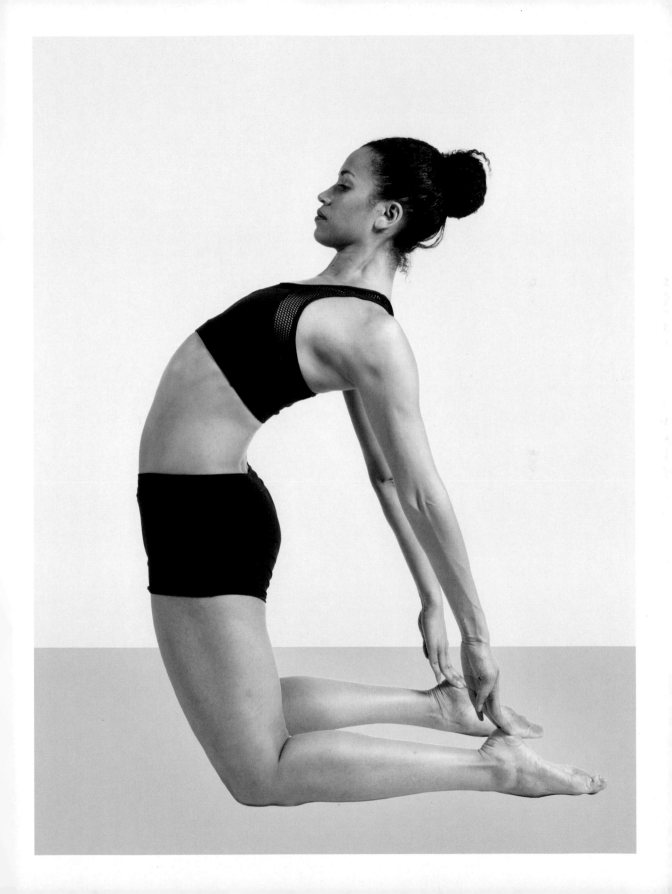

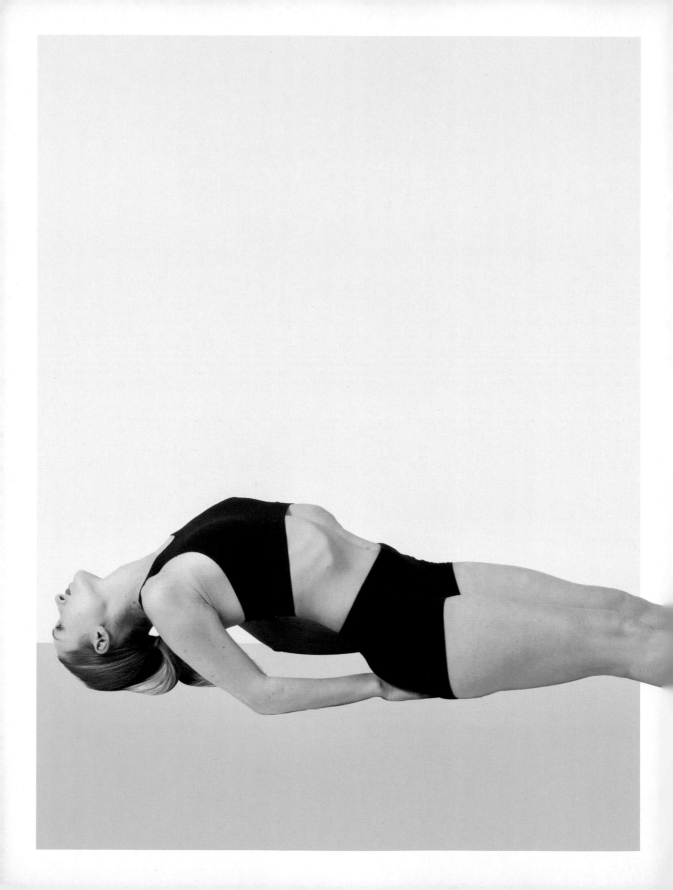

Fish Pose

The intermediate pose known as MATSYASANA in Sanskrit stretches the neck, chest, abdomen, and hip flexors along with the intercostal muscles of your ribs. It also strengthens the upper back and neck. Fish Pose is often paired with Shoulderstand.

FIND YOUR FORM
Keep your abdominal muscles taut to help support your lower back.

BE CAREFUL OF...
Do not let your torso droop into your lower back. Avoid this pose if you have isses with your neck or lower back.

STEPS
1. Begin lying faceup with your arms at your sides, knees bent, feet on the floor.
2. Slide your hands under your buttocks, and ease your hips up off the mat.
3. Bring your shoulder blades together, and press down with your palms, forearms, and elbows as you lift your back and shoulders off the mat in a hollow arc.
4. Tip your head back until your crown in on the mat; straighten both legs, toes pointed.
5. Internally rotate your thighs and press down as you stretch into the balls of your feet. Hold for three to five breaths.

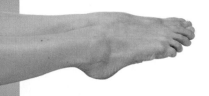

VARIATIONS
Therapeutic Fish: By placing a yoga block under your thoracic spine and umder your head, you can turn this pose into a restorative backbend.
Legs Elevated: To increase the intensity, while in hold, raise both extended legs up off the mat while maintaining form with your torso.

BEGINNER
INTERMEDIATE
ADVANCED

Bed Pose

FIND YOUR FORM
Be sure to engage your abdominal muscles and lower back muscles as you arch up and into the backbend.

BE CAREFUL OF...
Avoid this pose is you suffer from low-back, knee, or neck issues.

Also known as Couch Pose or PARYANKASANA, this relaxing position is effective for fostering better sleep patterns—if performed before bedtime it will soon have you deep in dreamland. This intermediate pose opens up the hips as well as extending the upper back and the shoulders.

STEPS

1. Begin by kneeling low on the mat, buttocks on the ground, with your hips alongside your feet. Your soles should be face up, with your feet alongside your hips.
2. Place your hands flat on the floor behind your hips. One at a time, lower your arms so that you are resting on your elbows and forearms.
3. Slowly ease your head back and touch the top of your head to the floor. Lift your elbows from the floor and place your hands on your hips.
4. Allow your spine to entend throughout its length as you hold the pose for four to six breaths.

VARIATION
Arms Entwined Bed Pose: From Bed Pose bring your arms over your head and rest your bent forearms on the floor, stacked sideways above your brow. Cup the opposite elbow with each hand.

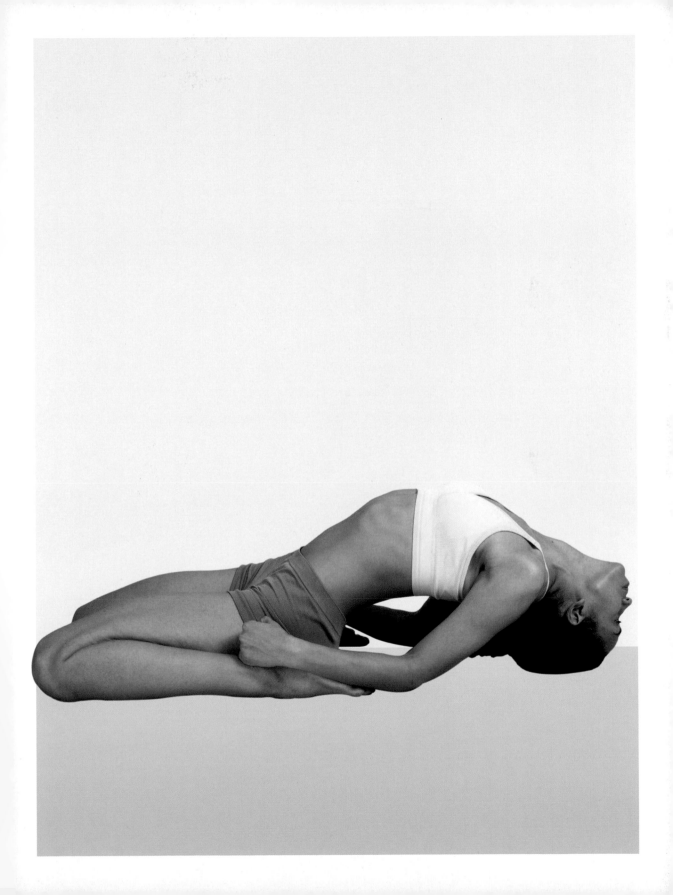

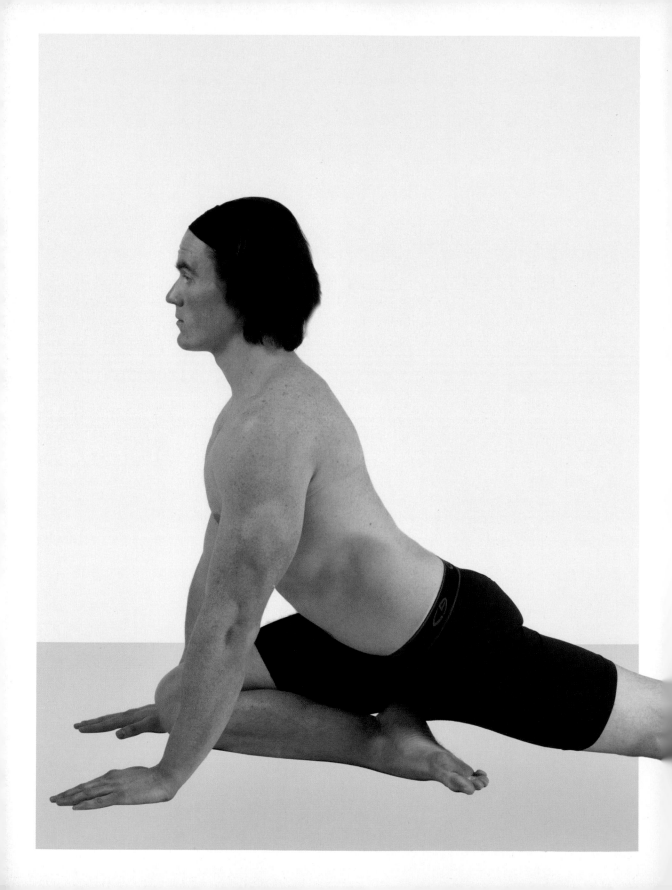

BEGINNER
INTERMEDIATE
ADVANCED

One-Legged King Pigeon Prep

FIND YOUR FORM

Your weight should primarily rest on your bent leg. Engage your abdominals muscles to protect your lower back as you puff up your chest...like a pigeon.

BE CAREFUL OF...

Avoid this pose if you suffer from groin or hamstring injuries.

Before advancing into the truly challenging One-Legged King Pigeon poses, try this prep pose. This asana will stretch the lower body and upper legs as well as opening the chest and shoulders. It makes a very good pose on its own to ease stress, anxiety, and fatigue.

STEPS

1. Begin kneeling on the mat, your buttocks positioned on your heels, your arms at your sides.
2. Extend your right leg behind you, with the top of your foot on the mat, toes facing back. Be sure to keep your bent knee facing straight forward.
3. Reach forward with both arms and place your hands, palms down just in front of your bent knee. Maintain a slight bend in the elbows.
4. Slide your left foot beneath your right hip as you tuck your pubis down and create a gentle arch in your lower back.
5. With your gaze forward, hold for three to six breaths before switching sides.

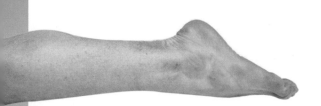

VARIATION

Prop Aid: You can place a yoga block under the bent leg in order to keep the hips square, which will align the lumbar spine and reduce the chance of strain on your joints.

BEGINNER
INTERMEDIATE
ADVANCED

One-Legged King Pigeon

The One-Legged King Pigeons are a group of advanced backbends that puff up the chest, like a strutting pigeon. The basic pose, EKA PADA RAJAKAPOTASANA, is a powerful hip opener that aids digestion and increases flexibility and range of motion in the spine and shoulders.

FIND YOUR FORM

Be sure to keep your hips squared to the front and your rear knee centered. Sit deeply into the pose, grounding your pubis.

BE CAREFUL OF…

If your chest or shoulders are tight, don't compensate by crunching your lower back. Avoid this pose if you have a hip, back, or knee injury.

STEPS

1. Begin in One-Legged King Pigeon Pose Prep, with your right leg behind you, knee centered, your left foot tucked under your right hip, and your hands planted in front of you.
2. Sit fully upright, pressing down with your fingertips and your pubic bone and hips to elevate your upper torso.
3. Bend your extended right leg, bringing your foot up, toes pointed, so that your heel moves toward your buttocks.
4. With your right elbow facing the ceiling, reach past your head, palm up, and grasp your raised toes on the outside of your foot. Ease your head back and reach past your head with your left hand to grasp your toes. Draw your foot gently toward your crown.
5. With your chin pointing up and your gaze on the ceiling, hold for three to five breaths before switching sides.

VARIATION

Lower Toe Hold: For less of an extreme backbend, after Step 3, while supporting your torso with your outstretched left hand, reach straight back behind you with your right hand to grasp the inside of your raised foot. Your back elbow should be bent and your right shin should be perpendicular to the floor.

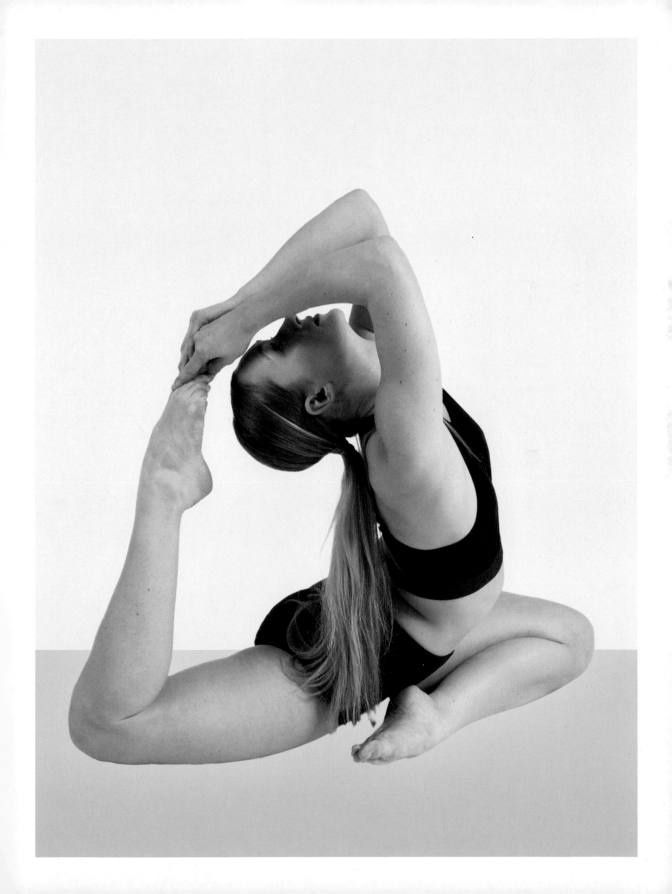

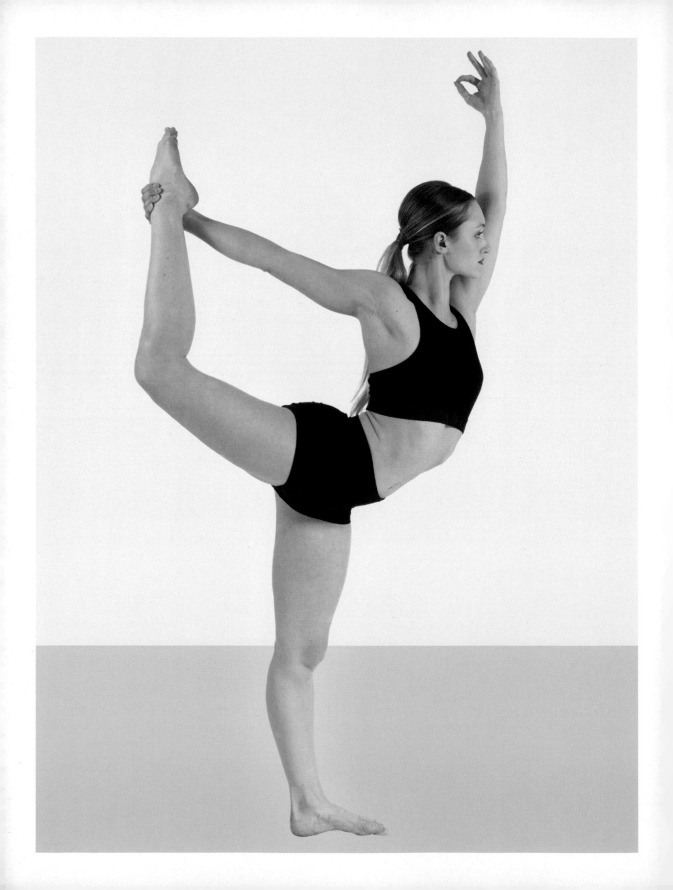

BEGINNER

INTERMEDIATE

ADVANCED

Lord of the Dance Pose

NATARAJASANA is a classic advanced yoga pose that not only requires flexibility of the legs, hips, shoulders, and back, it asks that you balance on one leg. It may be a demanding pose, yet it can be worked on incrementally, so that it is not beyond the reach of any level student.

FIND YOUR FORM

Be sure to stretch up through your forward arm and back through your raised leg before attempting the complete backbend. Keep your standing leg straight, with the muscles contracted.

BE CAREFUL OF...

If you feel wobbly at first, perform the pose facing a wall and place your raised hand on it for support. Avoid this pose if you have a back injury or low blood pressure.

STEPS

1. Begin standing in Mountain Pose (p.16). Bend your right knee, and raise your foot up with the heel moving toward your buttocks.
2. With your right palm facing outward, reach back and grasp the inside of your raised foot with your right hand.
3. Elevate your spine from tailbone to neck as you raise your left arm up, palm facing in, thumb and forefinger in a circle—the gyan mudra.
4. Raise your back foot toward the ceiling as you press it against your right hand. There should be extension in both arms and both legs and openness in your shoulders, chest, and groin. Your torso should remain as upright as possible without compressing your back.
5. With your gaze forward, hold for three to five breaths before switching sides.

VARIATION
Wide-Leg Lord of the Dance: More advanced students may want to try straightening the raised leg as much as is comfortable into a sort of aerial split.

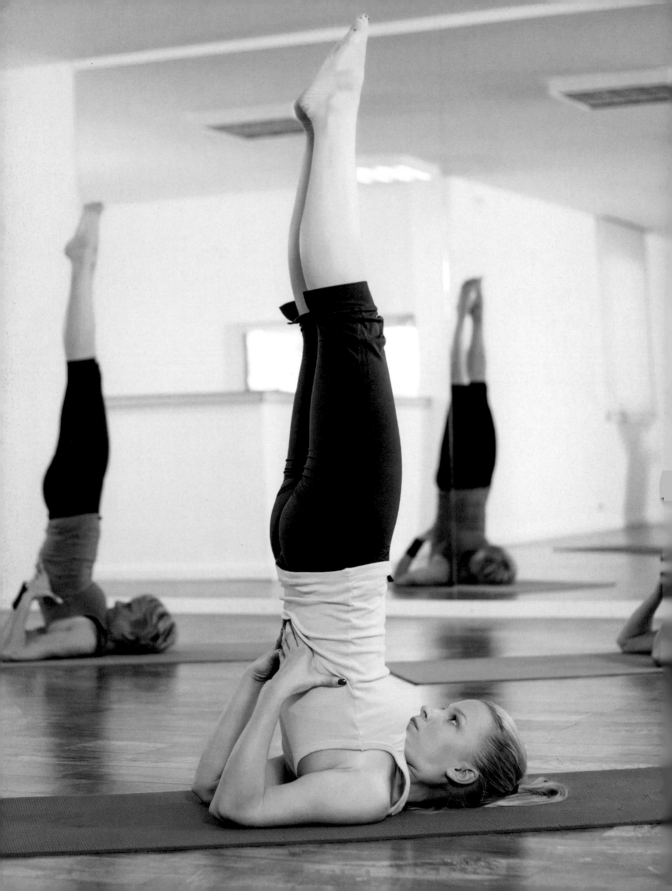

CHAPTER SEVEN

Inversions

Inversions are balance poses that reverse the effects of gravity and conclude with the heart positioned higher than the head. This makes them excellent for improving circulation, especially to the brain, as well as clearing congested sinuses and lungs. These poses utilize the abdominal muscles as stabilizers and strengthen the upper body. They are also known to offer psychological benefits, even helping to relieve depression and anxiety.

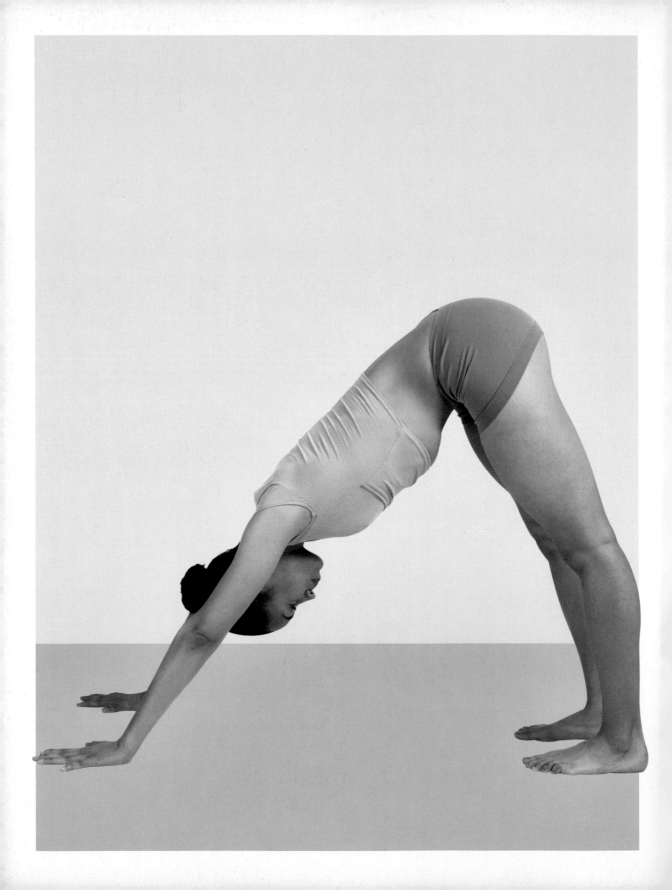

Downward-Facing Dog

FIND YOUR FORM

Place your weight on your outstretched hands rather than your wrist. Your lowered head should be in line with your spine, which should not be rounded.

BE CAREFUL OF...

Do not hold your breath; be sure to keep your jaw relaxed as you take normal breaths. Avoid this pose if you have shoulder or hamstring issues, carpal tunnel syndrome, or low blood pressure.

This well-known beginner asana, also called ADHO MUKHA SVANASANA, may look fairly simple, but it works most of the body, including strengthening the arms and legs, and stretching the spine, glutes, hamstrings, calves, and the arches of your feet.

STEPS

1. Begin down on all fours, with your hands positioned directly below your shoulders, palms down, and your knees below your hips.
2. Curl your toes forward as you walk your hands five to seven inches in front of your shoulders.
3. Ground your toes and palms into the mat as you raise your hips, eventually straightening your legs and planting your heels on the floor.
4. Draw your chest toward your thighs, and lower your head until it is positioned between your outstretched arms. Lengthen your spine at the tailbone, and internally rotate your thighs slightly, seeking a neutral pelvis.
5. With your gaze straight back or on your navel, hold for three to six breaths.

VARIATION

One-Legged Dog: While in hold, raise one leg to hip height with the foot flexed. Revolved Downward-Facing Dog: While in hold, swivel your shoulders as you reach your left hand back to the outside of the opposite foot, then switch hands.

BEGINNER
INTERMEDIATE
ADVANCED

Dolphin Pose

FIND YOUR FORM

Your back should remain straight throughout the pose; if this becomes painful, slightly bend your knees.

BE CAREFUL OF...

Do not raise your heels off the mat while in hold. Avoid this pose if you have neck or back injuries, a headache, or high blood pressure.

Dolphin Pose, also known as ARDHA PINCHA MAYURASANA, is very effective for building both strength and stability—it strengthens the shoulder girdle, improves your forearm stand and headstand, tones the abdominals, and, like other inversions that ask you to lower your head, it builds confidence.

STEPS

1. Begin down on all fours, arms positioned below your shoulders, knees below your hips.
2. Lower your forearms to the mat.
3. Raise your sit bones into the air as you straighten both legs. Bring your heels to the floor. Draw your tailbone toward your pubis, and squeeze your legs together.
4. Press into your forearms as you extend the stretch downward through your upper torso and shoulders; keep your head and chest off the floor.
5. While gazing backward hold for four to eight breaths.

VARIATIONS

Dolphin Split: While in hold, raise one leg until it is aligned with your torso, toes pointed.

Clasped Hands: Before elevating your hips, anchor your elbows under your shoulders, then clasp your hands together in front of you.

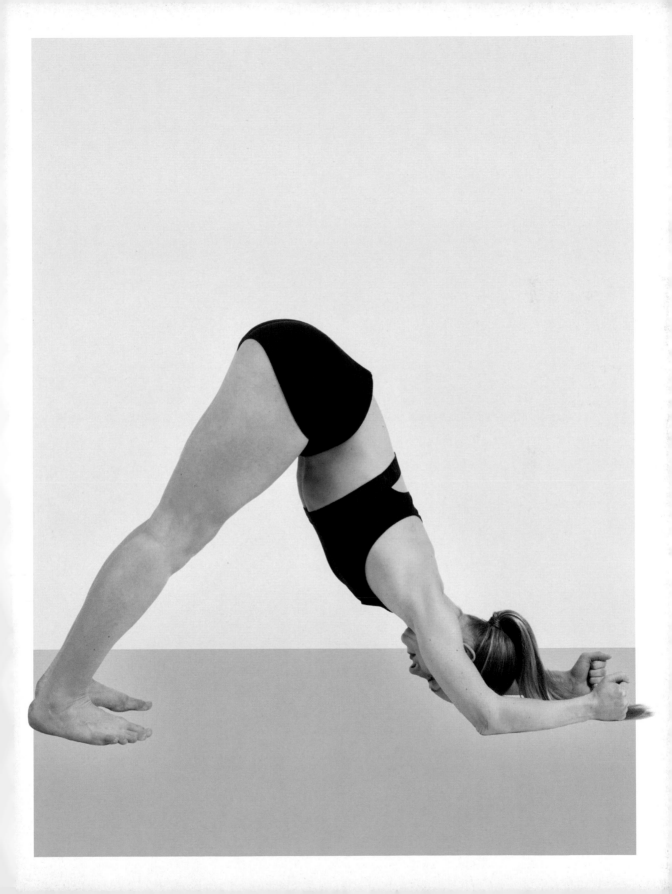

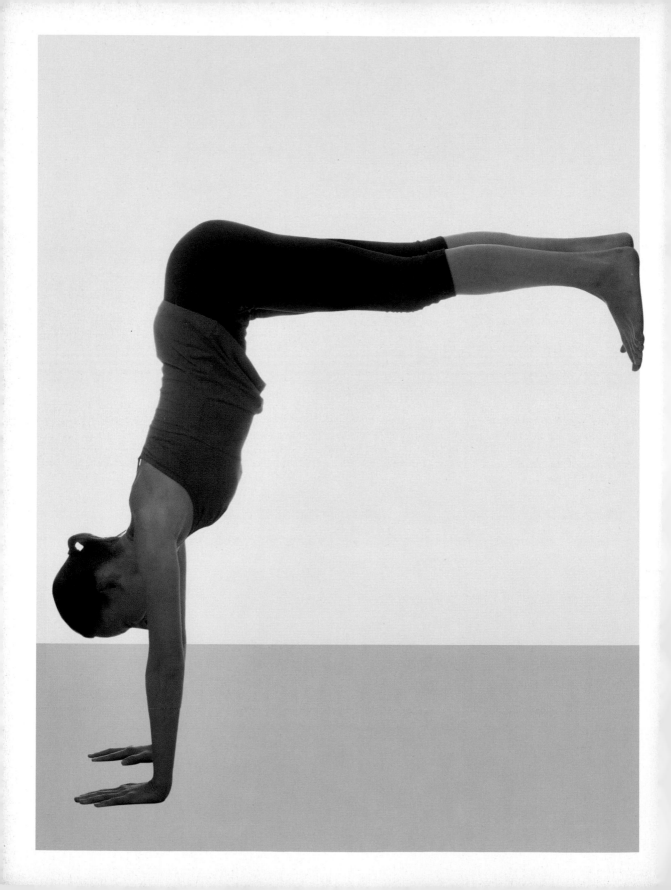

BEGINNER
INTERMEDIATE
ADVANCED

"L" at the Wall

This pose is accessible to students of all levels and makes a great prep for doing handstands. It works the muscles of the chest, upper arms, abdomen, sides, thighs, and buttocks, while it challenges your sense of balance and ability to distribute your weight.

FIND YOUR FORM

Keep your tailbone pushing up toward the ceiling. Your neck should remain in neutral position. For better stability, try carrying your weight over the roots of your fingers.

BE CAREFUL OF...

Avoid this pose if you have wrist issues or feel any pain in that area during the lift.

STEPS

1. Begin on all fours in tabletop position, palms down, with your feet at an unobstructed wall.
2. While externally rotating your arms and drawing your navel toward your spine, raise your hips into a Downward-Facing Dog with your heels right at the wall.
3. Carefully walk your feet up the wall until your heels align with your hips, and your body has formed an L shape.
4. Continue to stabilize your back by externally rotating your upper arms and tucking your abdomen in.
5. With your gaze on the floor, hold for three to six breaths. Lower one foot and then the other; fold down into Child's Pose.

VARIATION

One-Legged: To increase the difficulty level, once you feel stable, raise one leg toward the ceiling.

BEGINNER
INTERMEDIATE
ADVANCED

Supported Shoulder Stand

FIND YOUR FORM

Keep your throat soft and your tongue relaxed. If your neck protests, place a folded blanket under your shoulders.

BE CAREFUL OF...

Avoid bending your hips once you are in hold; that will place added pressure on your neck or spine. Also keep your elbows from splaying out. Avoid this pose if you have neck issues, a headache or ear infection, or high blood pressure.

This hatha yoga pose, SALANGA SARVANGASANA in Sanskrit, has many variations and is often called the "queen" or "mother" of asanas. This version may look intimidating but it is well within the scope of an intermediate-level student. It stretches the shoulders, neck, and upper back, and increases balance.

STEPS

1. Begin lying on your back with your knees bent, arms relaxed at your sides.
2. On an exhale, tighten your abdominals, press down with your arms, and raise your legs into the air enough so that your buttocks are lifted.
3. Continuing the arm pressure, bring your legs over your head, knees moving toward your face, as you roll your hips and back off the mat. Bend your elbows, and press your hands to your lower back. Keep your elbows tucked close to your sides.
4. Draw your tailbone toward your pubis, and align your legs again over your head until your torso is perpendicular to the floor and resting on your shoulders.
5. Inhale and consciously extend your legs toward the ceiling, opening your hips as you squeeze your buttocks and press the mat with your elbows.
6. With your gaze on the ceiling, hold for three to five breaths, then ease down to the mat.

VARIATION

Wall Walk: If the pelvic lift is hard at first, you can practice this pose a few feet from a wall; walk your feet up the wall and then place your hands against your lower back.

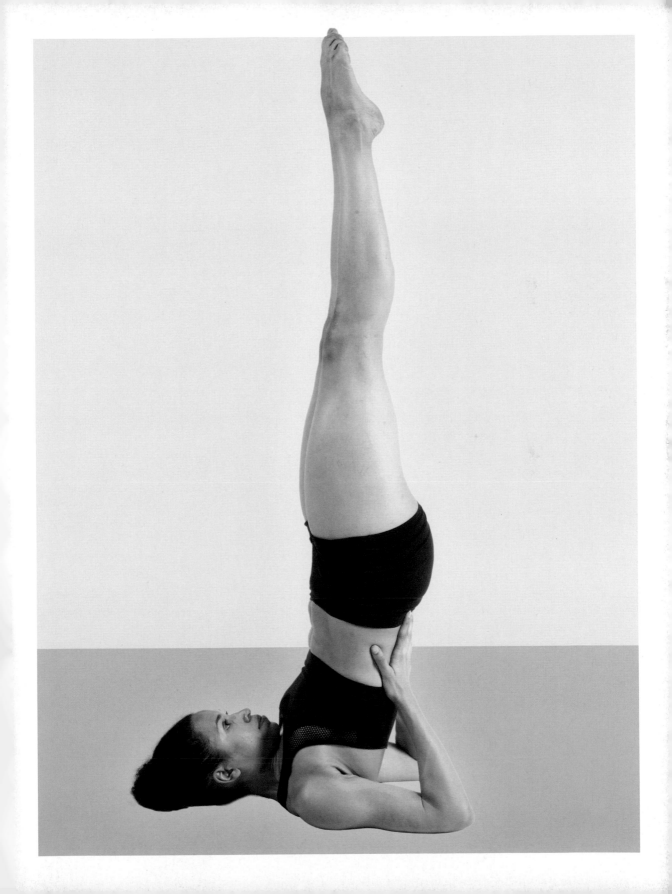

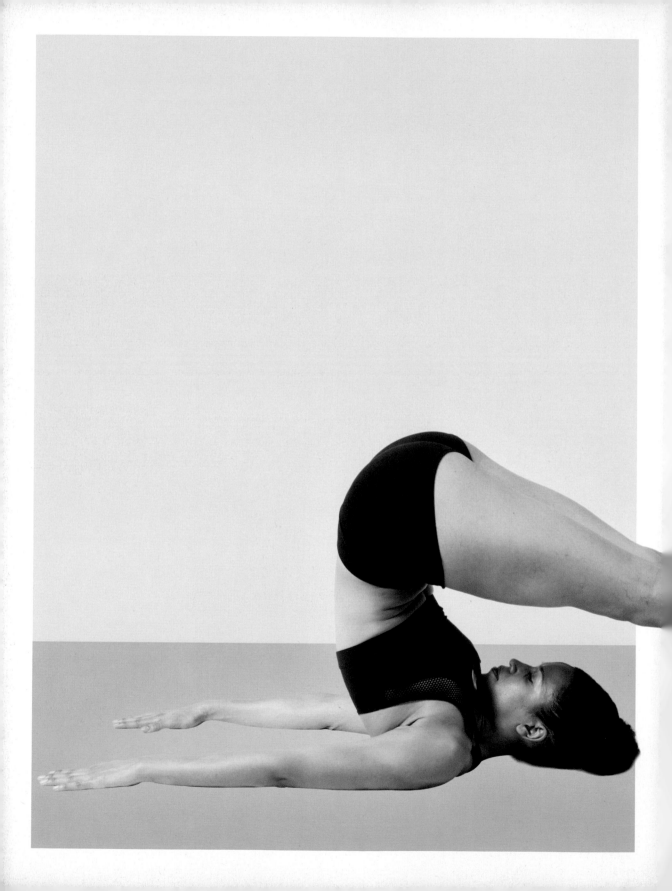

BEGINNER
| INTERMEDIATE |
ADVANCED

Plow Pose

FIND YOUR FORM
Make sure to keep your throat soft, Use a folded blanket under your shoulders if your nek protests. Keep your legs straight while in hold.

BE CAREFUL OF...
Don't use the weight of your legs to swing them down into the final position; lower them with control. Avoid this pose if you have neck issues, high blood pressure, or are pregnant.

This intermediate inversion, also known as HALASANA, stretches the entire back of the body, from heels to shoulders. It is considered a rejuvenating pose, one that soothes and restores the sympathetic nervous system, improves memory, and relieves stress. Plow Pose is also found in a number of yoga sequences.

STEPS
1. Begin by lying on your back with your knees bent, arms at your sides, palms down.
2. While tightening your abdomen, raise your legs straight up off the mat.
3. On an inhale, press down on your arms and shoulders and draw your tailbone toward your pubis as you begin to roll your lower torso off the mat. Begin with your buttocks, then your hips, and finally your back...until your legs are over your head. Your torso should be perpendicular to the floor.
4. On an exhale, allow your legs to extend farther over your head; squeeze them together, and bend at the waist until your tiptoes can touch the floor behind your head. By pressing into the mat with your arms and palms, you will continue to lift your hips.
5. With your gaze upward, hold for three to five breaths before easing down to the mat.

VARIATIONS
Back Support: For an easier lift, place both hands on your lower back as you roll up.
Intense Back Stretch: To increase the challenge, bring your arms straight back from your shoulders, and reach for your toes.

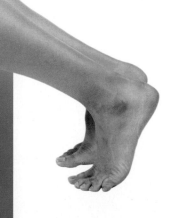

BEGINNER

INTERMEDIATE

ADVANCED

Supported Head Stand

FIND YOUR FORM

In final hold, support your weight evenly between your two forearms. If you can't keep your back straight—if its sags or rounds—try bending your knees slightly.

BE CAREFUL OF...

Do not allow your forehead to rest on the floor; this could cause compression in your neck. Do not jump up into the pose or kick up into the pose one leg at a time. Avoid this pose if you have back or neck issues, high blood pressure, or suffer from glaucoma.

This advanced pose, called SALAMBA SIRSASANA in Sanskrit, is also known to enthusiasts as the "king of asanas." It works the back, shoulders, and sides, while it offers clarity of mind, relieves stress, improves circulation, and aids digestion.

STEPS

1. Begin down on all fours, arms shoulder-width apart; place your forearms on the mat.
2. Externally rotate your outer upper arms and interlace your fingers, creating a cradle for your head. Raise your hips, straighten your legs, and tuck your toes under as you transition into Dolphin Pose.
3. Ease your fingers apart slightly as you place your crown on the mat and rest the back of your head against your entwined hands.
4. Press your forearms down as you lift your heels from the ground, and walk your feet toward your head until your hips are above your shoulders. Press your chest toward your thighs to help you raise your torso and protect your neck.
5. Bend one knee into your chest, then the other. As your balance stabilizes, begin raising both legs together toward the ceiling. Slightly rotate your thighs internally and lengthen your tailbone toward your feet. Keep the back of your legs and your glutes active.
6. Hold this upright position for three to five breaths before folding down into Child's Pose.

VARIATIONS

Wall Aid: If you have trouble maintaining your balance in hold, practice the pose with your shoulders supported against a wall.
Jackknife Stand: In final hold, angle your hips slightly behind your shoulders and fold both legs down until they are parallel to the floor.

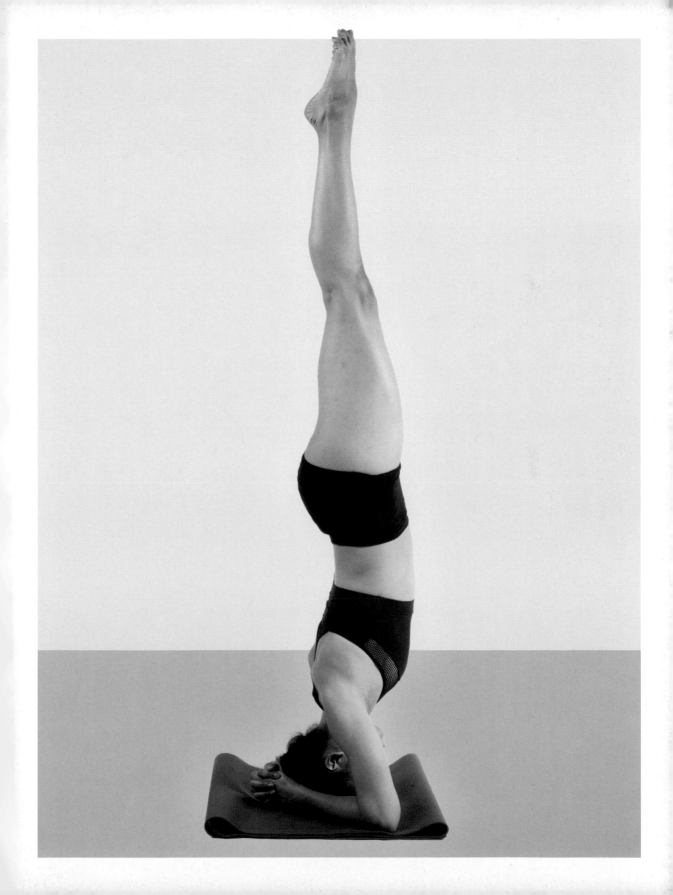

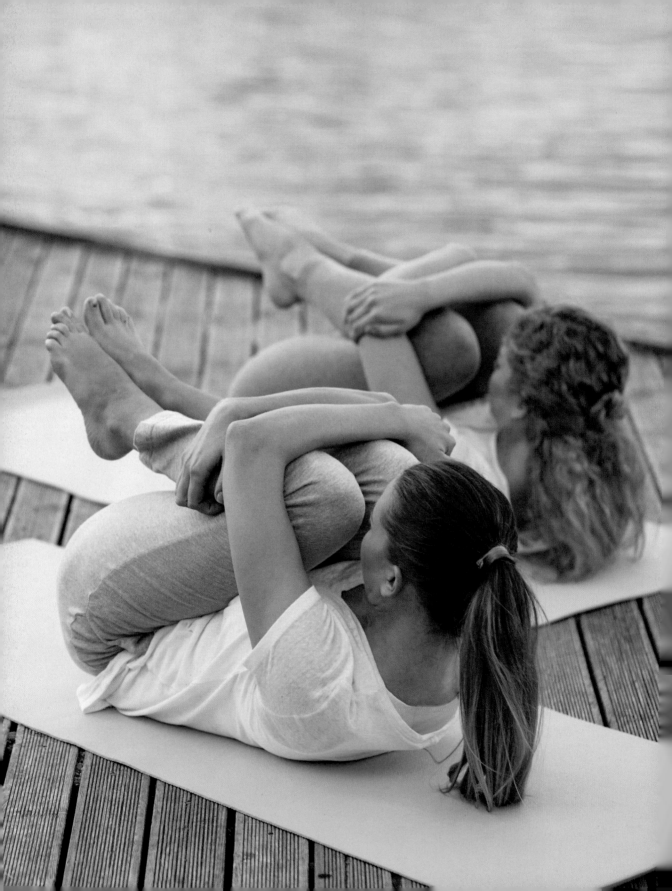

CHAPTER EIGHT

Reclining Poses

Reclining poses are a key element of restorative yoga that allow you to reset both mind and body. Supine poses, those where you lie on your back, help release stress and promote flexibility. They also make an excellent way to end a yoga session, allowing the student to cool down while benefiting from a powerful, uplifting sense of well-being.

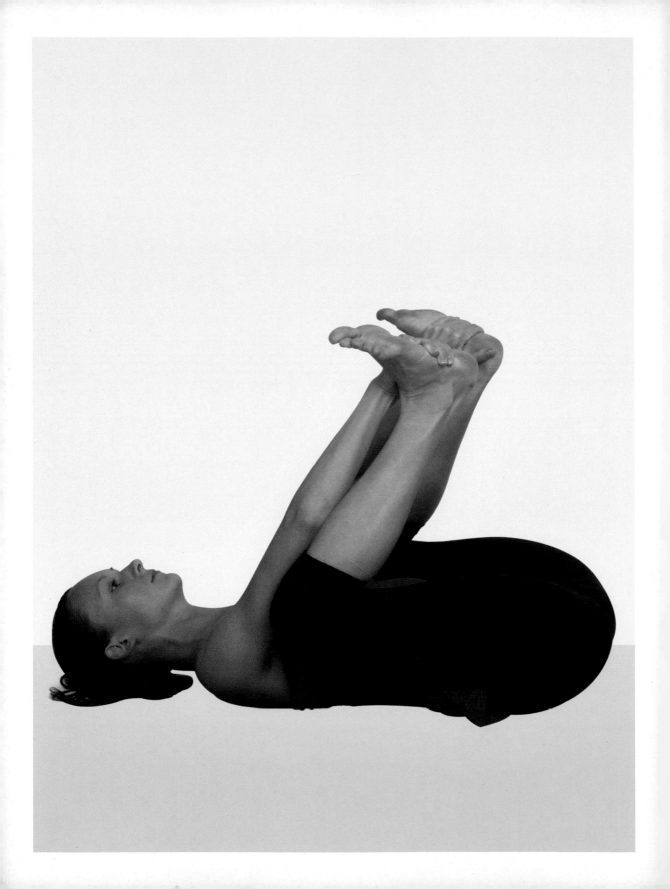

BEGINNER
INTERMEDIATE
ADVANCED

Happy Baby

FIND YOUR FORM

Tuck your pelvis forward a bit; this engages your abdominals and anchors your lower back. Keep your elbows bent slightly, and roll your shoulders forward off the mat.

BE CAREFUL OF...

Do not allow your head or shoulder blades to rise off the mat. Avoid this pose if you have lower-back issues or a groin injury.

This popular beginner pose is often used as part of a warm-up or cool-down session. It opens the hips and extends the muscles across the lower back, while stretching the stretching the glutes, hamstrings, and calves.

STEPS

1. Begin by lying flat on your back with your legs bent and your feet on the mat.
2. Raise both feet from the floor and draw your knees in toward your chest. Your soles should be facing the ceiling.
3. Reach up with both hands and take hold of the inside edges of your feet.
4. Gently pull down on your feet until your thighs are beside your sides and parallel to the floor.
5. Gaze up at the ceiling while holding this pose for four to eight breaths.

VARIATION

Crossover Baby: While in Happy Baby Pose, release your soles, cross your arms and grasp the opposite inside ankles

Reclining Spinal Twist

FIND YOUR FORM

Be sure to keep your elbows and wrists slightly lower than your shoulders to protect your rotator cuffs.

BE CAREFUL OF...

Do not hunch your shoulders up around your ears; both shoulder blades should remain flat on the mat. Avoid this pose if you have hip issues or a lower-back injury.

VARIATIONS

Head Twist: To add a stretch to your neck, when in hold turn your face and gaze away from the side with the bent knee.

Knee Hold: For a more demanding pose, place your left palm on the quad of the crossed-over right leg, and vice versa.

Also known as SUPTA MATSYENDRASANA in Sanskrit, this beginner pose comprises a spinal twist that increase mobility in the back and helps to relieve tension. It also stretches the outer hips and glutes while massaging the internal organs.

STEPS

1. Begin lying faceup on the mat, legs parallel, arms outspread slightly below your shoulders, palms up.
2. Bend your right knee, raise your leg off the mat, and cross it over your body while rotating your hips so that your right buttock is also raised up. Your upper torso should remain flat on the floor.
3. With your torso and extended leg forming a straight line, lower your right knee to the mat beyond your hips; your thigh should be at a right angle to your body.
4. Gaze upward, and hold for four to eight breaths before repeating on the other side.

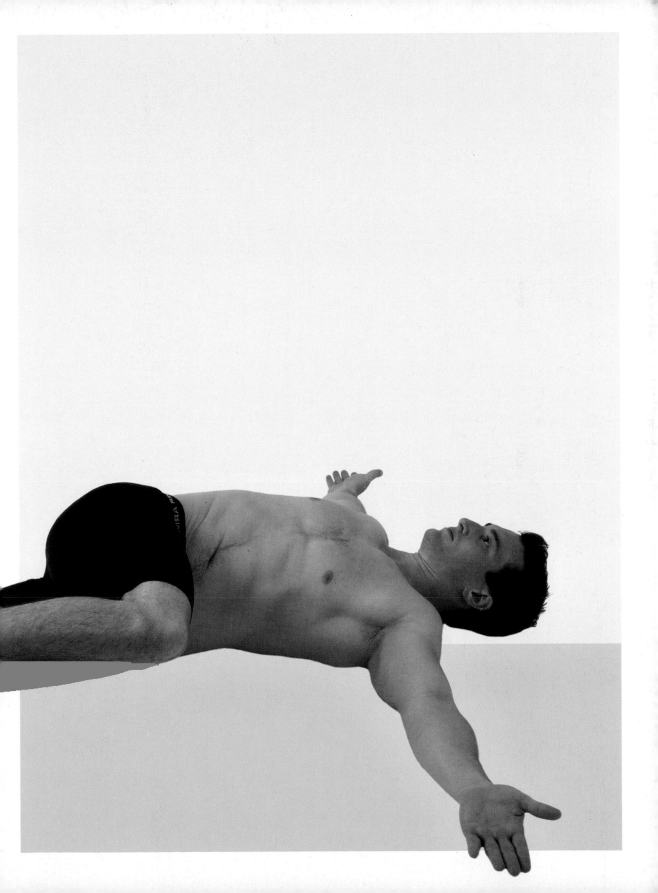

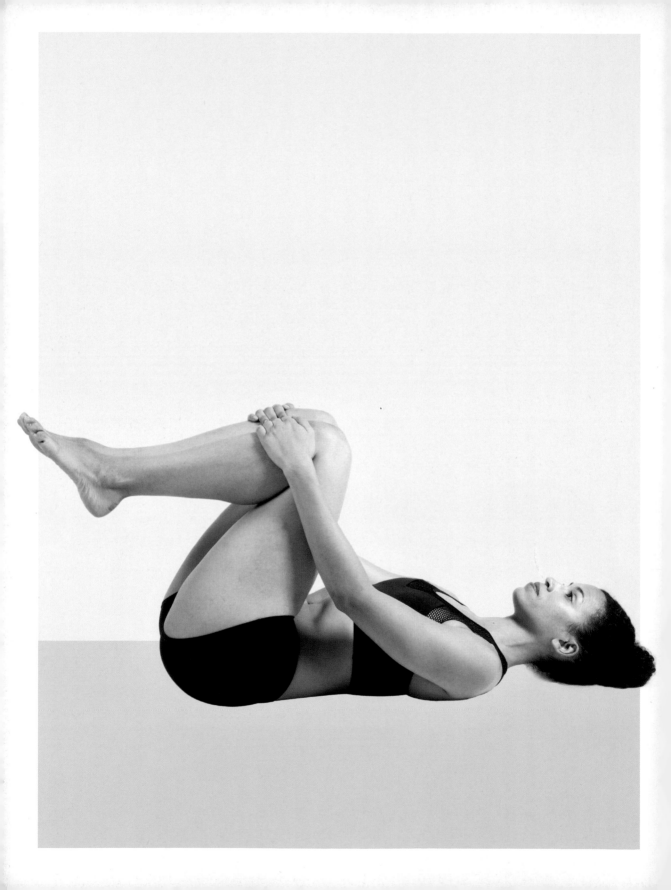

BEGINNER

BEGINNER

INTERMEDIATE

ADVANCED

Knees-to-Chest Pose

Known as APANASANA in Sanskrit, this relaxing beginner pose provides excellent therapy for lower-back pain caused by tension or stress. It also opens the hips, tones the glutes and hamstrings, massages the internal organs, and eases digestive complaints.

FIND YOUR FORM

Make sure your hips remain on the floor as you raise your legs. Keep your neck in neutral position, and angle your chin away from your chest.

BE CAREFUL OF...

While holding the pose, do not tense your leg or back muscles. Avoid this pose if your are pregnant or have a knee injury.

STEPS

1. Begin lying faceup with your legs extended on the mat.
2. On an exhale, raise both knees and bring them toward your chest until your shins are parallel to the floor.
3. Grasp your shins just below the knees with both hands. Keep your shoulder blades flat on the mat as you pull your knees in closer.
4. Consciously lengthen your tailbone as you elongate your spine, and flatten your back and shoulders on the floor.
5. With your gaze on the ceiling, hold for four to eight breaths.

VARIATIONS

Single Knee: You can practice the pose by holding only one knee to your chest at a time; keep the other leg extended, foot flexed.

Elbow Touch: For more intensity, wraps your arms around your knees and grasp the opposite elbow with each hand.

Wind-Relieving Pose

FIND YOUR FORM

Your navel should be tucked toward your spine to stabilize your core; keep the middle and upper back flat against the mat.

BE CAREFUL OF...

If you feel pain when holding your neck up, place a folded blanket under your head. Avoid this pose if you have hip or groin issues or low-back pain.

This therapeutic reclining pose, also known as PAVANA MUKTASANA, is especially effective for treating the cramping and pain of intestinal gas. It opens the lower back and tones the abdominal muscles while stretching the neck, thighs, and glutes.

STEPS

1. Begin in Knees-to-Chest Pose (p.210) with your hips on the mat and your knees drawn toward your chest, feet flexed.
2. On an exhale, roll your lower torso up until your buttocks and hips are off the mat.
3. Cross your hands over your shins, and draw your knees toward you until your thighs are resting against your chest.
4. Angle your head up off the mat until you are gazing at your knees.
5. Hold for three to six breaths.

VARIATION

One-Legged: Keep your left leg extended on the mat while hugging the bent right leg at the top of the shin. Draw your thigh against your chest.

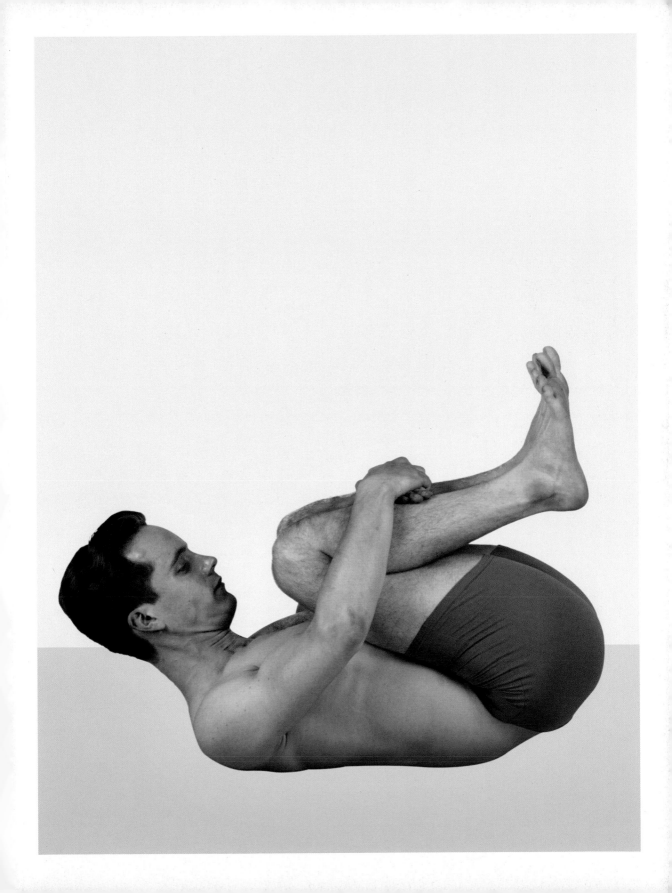

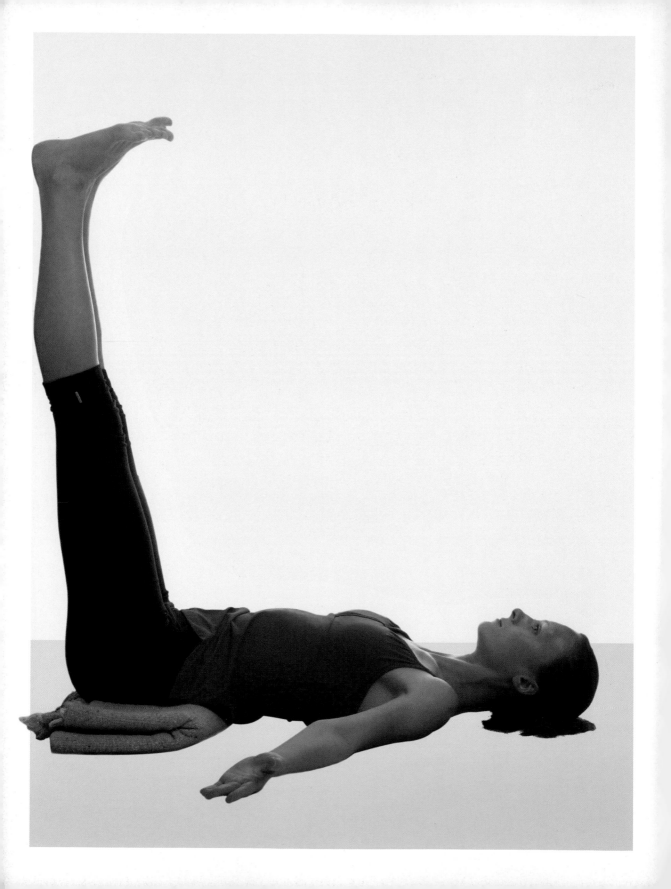

INTERMEDIATE
ADVANCED

Legs Up the Wall

FIND YOUR FORM

Your arms may be outspread or positioned along your body; press down to provide a stable base. Gravity will naturally lower your legs into your pelvis and release your back and head into the floor.

BE CAREFUL OF...

Do not allow your abdomen or chest to sag. Avoid this pose if you have a headache or groin or hip issues.

This beginner pose, also known as VIPARITA KARANI, uses a wall to create a reclining inversion. While it may take some practice to get into the pose, it is a great way to work your abdominals, your glutes, and the backs of your thighs, the biceps femoris, or hamstrings.

STEPS

1. Begin sitting beside a wall, with your shoulders perpendicular to the wall and your knees tucked up to your chest.
2. Angle your torso sideways away from the wall, and lie down as you raise your bent legs and swing them gently up against the wall.
3. Scoot your buttocks as close to the wall as possible as you extend your legs upward and flex your feet. Rest your heels against the wall.
4. With your neck in neutral position, hold for four to eight breaths.

VARIATION

Prop Aid: If you have difficulty with this pose at first, try adding a folded blanket under your hips or your head. If your hamstrings are stiff, add another blanket under your hips or move several inches from the wall.

BEGINNER
INTERMEDIATE
ADVANCED

Reclining Hero

FIND YOUR FORM

Allow yourself to sink back into the recline; never force yourself into any pose. Keep your neck in neutral position, not lolling back, as you lower yourself down.

BE CAREFUL OF...

This pose can be hard on the knees, so make sure your legs are limbered up before attempting it. Do not allow your knees to raise off the mat in hold. Avoid this pose if you have knee, ankle, or back issues or are menstruating.

SUPTA VIRASANA is an intermediate reclining pose that offers a deep stretch for your thighs while it loosens your quads and opens the arches of your feet. It is also useful for stimulating digestion, and alleviating respiratory problems and the symptoms of arthritis.

STEPS

1. Begin in Hero Pose (p. 94), sitting comfortably with your knees bent and buttocks fully on the mat.
2. On an exhale, lean back and place your hands behind you for support. Lower yourself down onto your elbows.
3. Gradually recline your torso until you are lying on the mat. Keep your abdominal muscles taut to protect your lower back, and squeeze your knees together to keep them at hip width.
4. Fan your arms out from your sides, palms up, in a relaxed posture of acceptance.
5. Gaze upward, and hold the pose for three to five breaths.

VARIATION

Prop Aid: If you can sit upright in Hero Pose, but have trouble reclining, place folded blankets under your hips and head.

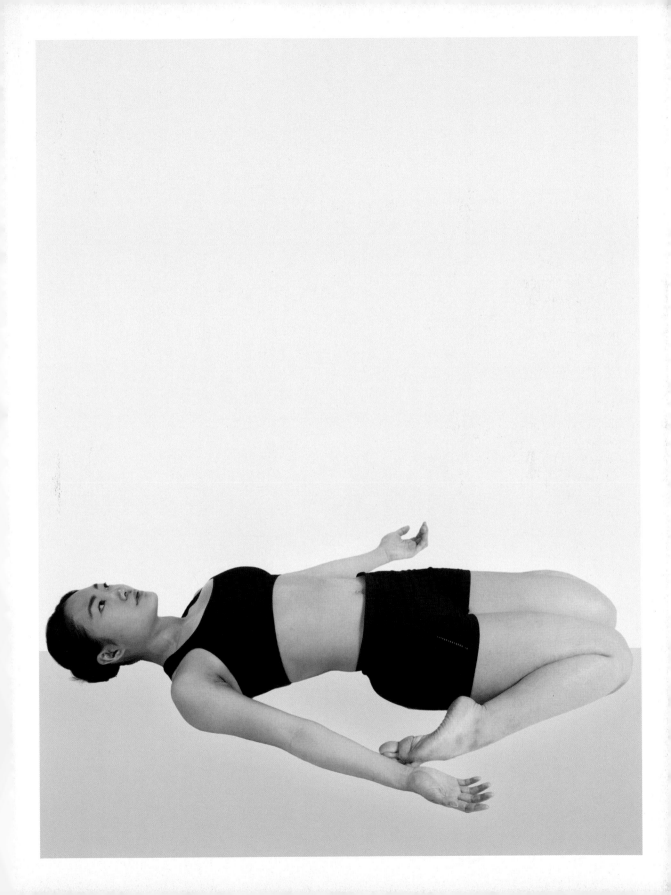

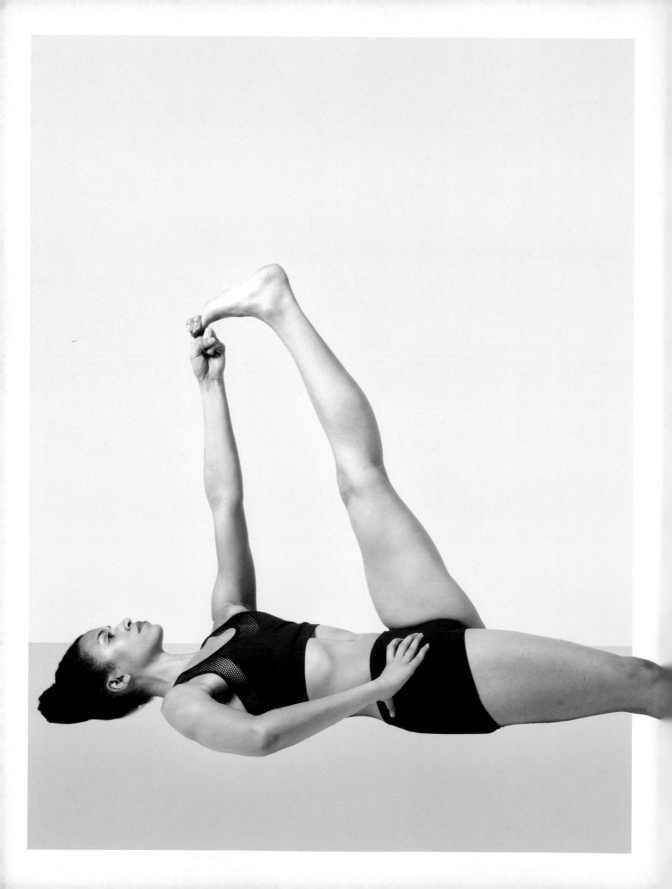

BEGINNER
INTERMEDIATE
ADVANCED

Reclining Big Toe Pose

FIND YOUR FORM

Keep your raised leg straight, and don't allow that hip to lift from the mat. Both your hips and buttocks should be deeply grounded.

BE CAREFUL OF...

This pose requires great flexibility; you might try it first with a yoga strap around your elevated foot. Avoid this pose after recent hip or knee surgery or if you have hamstring or groin issues.

This intermediate pose, called SUPTA PADANGUSTHASANA in Sanskrit, is a popular restorative asana that opens the groin and hips; stretches spine, hamstrings, and calves; and strengthens the knees and abdominals. Try this as a prep for more intense or challenging Big Toe Poses.

STEPS

1. Begin lying faceup on the mat, your legs extended.
2. Raise your left leg straight up until your heel is over your left hip...so that your left knee faces your armpit.
3. Reach up to your foot with your left hand, and wrap your forefinger and middle finger around the inside of your big toe.
4. Shift your whole leg to the left to increase the stretch to your hip and inner thigh; or draw it to the right to stretch your outer hip and IT band.
5. With your neck elongated and your gaze on the ceiling, hold for three to six breaths. Repeat on the other side.

VARIATION

Forehead Touch: For more challenge, roll your head and shoulders up from the mat, and use both hands to ease the shin of your raised leg toward your forehead... without bending your knee.

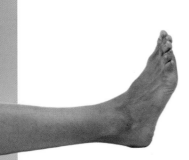

BEGINNER

INTERMEDIATE

ADVANCED

Corpse Pose

SAVASANA is often the final pose performed at the end of yoga class, allowing you to absorb the therapeutic benefits of your session. It can also relieve the fatigue caused by more demanding poses and induce calmness of mind. By remaining motionless and keeping your thoughts quiet, you can learn to truly relax. The pose also combats anxiety and depression and can help lower high blood pressure.

FIND YOUR FORM

It can help to imagine you are floating gently on a raft. Or feel the weight of your body and the presence of the ground supporting you, and then allow yourself to melt downward.

BE CAREFUL OF...

Do not allow yourself to fall asleep during Savasana. Avoid this pose if you have back issues.

VARIATIONS

Pentacle Pose: Extend your arms straight out to either side.

Constructive Rest Pose: Perform the pose with your knees bent; try adding a bolster under your back.

STEPS

1. Begin lying faceup on your back. Keep your legs wide apart, around the width of your mat, and let your feet roll open to the sides.
2. Bring your hands to your sides, away from your chest but not too far apart.
3. Relax completely, closing your eyes, softening all the muscles in your face and throat, and simply letting go. Breathe quietly and softly, gradually lengthening your exhales. Try not to fall asleep or let your mind wander—turn your gaze inward, and keep it there for about 5 to 10 minutes.
4. To emerge from Savasana, begin wiggling your fingers and toes, inhale and exhale deeply, draw your knees to your chest, and then roll to the side, taking pressure off the heart. Once you are alert again, you should feel completely re-energized and blissful.

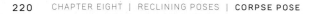

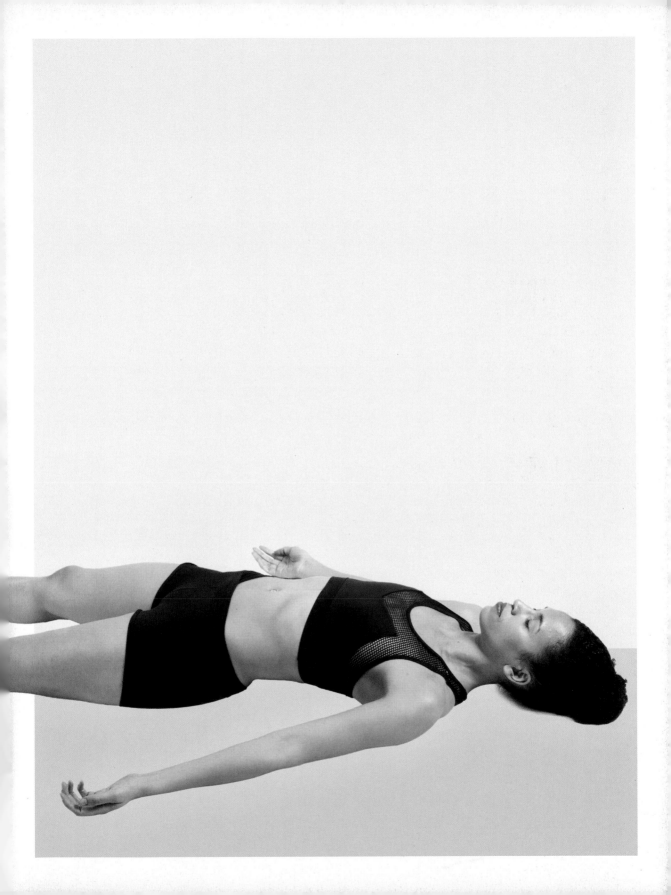

Glossary

Yoga incorporates many terms that are based on Sanskrit, the classical language of India, and which is found in ancient Hindu scriptures and epic poems. When these yoga terms are pronounced properly, distinct inhalations and exhalations occur that are similar to those used in meditative mantras.

Ashram
A monastic community or a religious retreat, especially in India and Southeast Asia.

Asana
A physical posture of yoga.

Ashtanga
The eight-limbed yogic path consisting of Yamas—ethical rules or moral imperatives; Niyama—virtuous habits, behaviors, and observances; Asana—postures; Pranayama—extended or controlled breathing; Pratyahara—drawing within one's awareness; Dharana—concentration, introspective focus; Dhyana—contemplation, reflection, profound abstract meditation; and Samadhi—oneness, joining, combining, harmonious whole.

Ayurveda
Ancient Indian science of health.

Bakasana
Sanskrit term for the basic Crane pose or Crow pose, where the folded torso is balanced above the arms and the bent knees rest upon bent elbows. Also called Kakasana.

Bakti
Devotion, as in Bakti yoga.

Bandha
An internal lock used for controlling the energy inside the body during yoga; the three locks practiced in Hatha yoga are the root lock, the abdominal lock, and the throat lock.

Buddha
The enlightened one; in Buddhism, refers to Siddhartha Gautama, an enlightened spiritual teacher during the sixth to fourth century BC.

Chakra
One of seven energy centers in the human body—root, sacrum, solar plexus, heart, throat, third eye, and crown. Each is associated with a color, element, syllable, significance, etc.

Dharma
Truth; the path of truth; the teachings of the Buddha.

Drishti
A gazing point or visual focus used during asanas.

Guru
Spiritual teacher or master; literally "one who illuminates the darkness".

Mantra
A repeated sound that facilitates the act of meditation; a sacred thought or prayer. Can be sounds, syllables, words, or groups of words that create a positive transformation.

Meditation
Focusing the mind through breath control in order to reach a deeper level of consciousness.

Mudra

A hand gesture used during asanas and meditation that influence one's energies. Palms are pressed together in prayer position, or anjali mudra, and forefinger and thumb touch in gyan mudra.

Namaste

"I bow to you," a greeting used between friends, or yoga instructors and students.

Om or Aum

Considered the first sound of creation, it is frequently chanted during meditation or before, during, or after yoga classes.

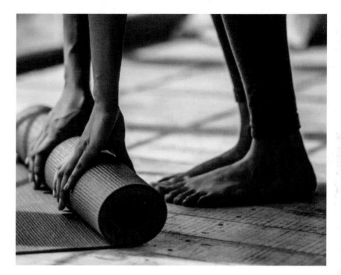

Prana

Life energy; chi; qi.

Pranayama

Breath awareness; control of breathing to improve mind/body connection.

Samadhi

A state of complete enlightenment.

Savasana

The Sanskrit term for Corpse Pose; typically, the final relaxation pose at the end of a yoga class.

Shakti

Female energy.

Shanti

Peace, the term is often chanted three time.

Shiva

Male energy; a Hindu deity.

Surya Namskar

Sun Salutations; a system of yoga poses performed in a series or flow.

Sutras

Classical Indian texts that systematized yogic principles.

Swami

Master, a Hindu ascetic or religious leader.

Tantra

The yoga of union between mind and body.

Yoga

From the Sanskrit yug or "to unite"; an ancient practice that incorporates breathing practices, physical postures, meditation, and philosophy in order to achieve enlightenment.

Yogi/Yogini

A male/female practitioner of yoga.

Acknowledgements

ABOUT THE AUTHOR

Nancy J. Hajeski is the author of nature, health, and wellness titles for publishers such as National Geographic, Thunder Bay, and Barnes & Noble. Recent books include the National Geographic titles: *Complete Guide to Herbs and Spices; Birds, Bees, and Butterflies; and Nature's Best Remedies.* Other health-related titles include *Essential Wellness, 501 Yoga Poses,* and *Ultimate Yoga.* She has also written home bartender guides *Mezcal: The Gift of the Agave* and *The Beer Handbook.* Nancy lives and works in the Catskill Mountains of New York.

PHOTOGRAPHY
Naila Ruechel
Jonathan Conklin

MODELS
Natasha Diamond-Walker
Larissa Terada
Jessica Gambelluri
Lloyd Knight
Daniel Wright
Goldie Oren
Lana Russo
Alex Geissbuhler
Roya Carreras
Conor Fallon
Alyssa Cebulski
Emilie Noelle
Kelly Jacobs

All other images © and courtesy of Shutterstock.and their contributors.
Picture research by Kate Williams at KatieLove Design Ltd.